Ketogenic Diet Cookbook

For Beginners

Two Weeks Meal Plan

for Weight Loss

By

Adam Sanders

Table of contents

Introduction

I am confident - it is more than mere chance you're holding this book in your hands. Perhaps, like I did, you came to Keto after a series of unsuccessful attempts to lose weight, a number of harassing diets, and countless attempts to become healthier and make your life a little bit better. You're almost desperate, aren't you? Don't give up! Let's follow some simple step-by-step tips. Following these useful rules can boost the quality of your life!

Before going deep into the basics of the diet, let me tell you how I have experienced the LCHF (low carbs, high fat) or Keto lifestyle. I'm motivating you into action!

My name is Adam. I celebrated my 35th birthday recently. Looking back, I thank fate for the accidental meeting 5 years ago that radically changed my life! But first things first.

By the age of 29, I have diseased knees, problem skin, and shortness of breath and am overweight (At a height of six feet, I weighed 250 pounds). As a present for my birthday, I received an annual gym membership. I decided to start a new life then!

The trainer came up with a training program and a personal nutrition plan (a diet with a minimum amount of fat, a large amount of proteins, and a low amount of carbs). During the first month of trainings, I lost ten pounds, and it was fantastic results! The only disadvantage was a constant desire to eat sweets. I didn't notice a desire before as I always have a neutral attitude to various kinds of cookies, sweets, and other delights.

However, I became obsessed with buying a package of cookies or a box of chocolates. In my dreams I pounced on showcases with cakes and pies eagerly swallowing them up one by one. With my experience, I understood that my brain was in desperate need of glucose, and the easiest way to get it was to eat fast carbs, like sugar.

Since then, sweets, all kinds of buns, and ice-cream appeared in my "diet". I allowed myself to eat a small cake on weekends! So despite my efforts in a gym, the loss of the weight stopped, and I just walked in circles. I was too irritable without sweets and often snapped at people around me. While buying sweets, I felt guilty, but I excused myself because of stress, troubles at work, etc.

I didn't know how long this struggle would continue, but at that time I finish reading Allen Carr's book, Easy Way to Stop Smoking. Finally, I decided to quit and successfully implemented the plan of improving my health. My life began to play with new colors;

tastes and smells became more intense, I had a new feeling of self-confidence and grew wings because I quit smoking!

But I gained weight. I took control of my diet by replacing the sweets with fruits and cutting out bread and pasta, but despite all these measures, I still weighed 270 pounds by my 30th birthday although my health, in general, was much better than the previous year.

The next period of my life I tried to be a vegetarian, but I only lasted two weeks. I can't imagine how vegetarians live without meat. Then I underwent the attempts of fasting. There was a periodic fasting, or as it is also called the food protocol sixteen by eight. You fast for sixteen hours, and during the next eight hours, you eat anything you want but staying within your daily calories.

After that I tried other various diets, which was the reduction of carbs and fats with a major focus on proteins. None of these variants worked because of my constant desire to eat something between meals. My thoughts wouldn't stop about eating, so I had to find the right solution that would help me not to focus on food all the time. Eventually, "we eat to live, and don't live to eat."

Apparently, the universe heard my requests, and at one of the trainings I met a new fitness club visitor, a wonderful girl Mary (my beloved wife now). She had the same problems as me. After she quit smoking, her weight and waist increased, and in addition, she faced hormone imbalance and fluid retention. There was only one difference between us. By the end of the second week, her transformation was noticeable, and in a month, she was a rather different person! I couldn't believe that such a transformation was possible without special additives and the latest achievements of sports pharmacology!

I made friends with Mary. She was the one who told me about Keto and how to lose fat by eating fat. I couldn't believe it! This information contradicted everything I knew before from advanced nutritionists, fitness gurus, and other people related to the food industry. After six months on Keto, I brought my weight back to a normal 183 pounds with my six feet height. I've gotten rid of feeling unwell. I no longer have a constant desire to eat, and the pain in my knees and skin problems are gone!

Today I'm not as strict in calculating calories. I don't eat according to the schedule, but when I want. I just try to get the most of energy from the right fats and to keep an amount of pure carbs to about fifty grams, not counting dietary fiber, per day. To represent the nutrients at a percentage, it will be approximately:

The amount of fats is seventy to seventy-five percent, proteins - twenty percent, carbohydrates - five to ten percent.

During a hard training, I am allowed to eat a banana.

If you're ready, I'd like to acquaint you with the Keto diet. You'll learn how to start using the diet. I'm going to tell you about what foods are allowed and what foods aren't. I'll share my favorite proven recipes with you. These recipes are ones I've tried myself.

Just one more "diet" or lifestyle?

Any diet is always perceived as something temporary, like some rules that need to be followed only at a certain time. Then, having achieved the planned results, we return to our normal ration. But we continue to restrict ourselves and count calories, secretly dreaming about a piece of cake or candy. The struggle you face is often accompanied by depression and nervous breakdowns. As a result, losing a couple of pounds doesn't make you happier. Many of us having tried Keto, including me, my wife and our friends, became followers of this diet. It has become a part of our lives!

The secret here is you shouldn't make enormous efforts to follow certain rules in nutrition. By eliminating carbs almost completely or limiting the consumption to a minimum of twenty-five to fifty grams per day, you can get the most of the daily calories from the right fats. It will cause you to feel good. There will no effect of a full stomach anymore, and the feel of hunger is gone. You start to understand your body better. You can change the time of your meals, and you can eat whenever you want. The amount of food is decreased. The process can be compared to coal at a power station, which would be replaced with nuclear fuel. There is a great efficiency with a small amount of fuel!

 The main task of a ketogenic diet is to set up your body for a new type of energy intake. You'll learn how to get the energy from fat, not from carbs like you used to do. Of course, you can also turn the body into a new regime with fasting, but it's big shoes. So, let's learn the basics of the Keto diet and consider each item step by step.

Ketosis

Ketosis is a metabolic state with a certain level of ketones (about 0.5 mmol / l). As a rule, people have a state of ketosis when they limit carbohydrates as much as possible (a result of a ketogenic diet) or don't eat at all (a result of several days of fasting). In general, the body won't launch ketosis if the diet contains enough carbs or stores glycogen, a form of sugar. to provide cells with an energy. Until the sugar is available, your body will use glucose as the main source of fuel. In fact, many people live their lives without entering ketosis and feel great.

If ketosis is not necessary to maintain optimal health, then there are a couple of questions: What is the purpose of the Keto diet? How do we feel about using fat and glucose as a fuel? In order to understand these issues better and to find out why we have the ability to use ketones as a fuel, we must consider two approaches: the health point of view and the evolution one.

Health

From the health point of view, ketones have a lot of unique properties in comparison with sugar. First, ketones are burned much more efficiently than sugar and provide us with a more productive source of energy forming the less reactive oxygen species. Ketones also increase the efficiency and productivity of mitochondrion, which greatly improves the ability of ketone cells to generate energy and to slow down aging. As a result of research, ketones are neuroprotective antioxidants that can stop brain damage during the process of generation of new brain cells and create links between already existing ones. As a result of the ketones burning, a shift happens in the balance between the two neurotransmitters called GABA and glutamate. Therefore, ketones contribute to the prevention of excessive neurons activity that can cause uncontrolled behavior, specific to some neurological disorders such as epilepsy, autism, and Parkinson's disease.

There is also a great amount of research confirming a ketogenic diet can improve some health conditions significantly.

In some cases, it can even help get rid of such diseases as:

Migraines

Fatty Liver Disease

Heart Disease

Polycystic Ovary Syndrome

Cancer

Obesity

Chronic Inflammation

High Blood Sugar Levels

Alzheimer's disease

Parkinson's disease

Type 2 Diabetes

Type 1 Diabetes

Epilepsy

Even if you don't have any of the diseases listed above, *using the diet you can have the following benefits:*

- An increase in energy - Better brain function

- A decrease in inflammation - Improved body composition

Evolutionary

Now let's find out why our body has the ability to enter the state of ketosis. From an evolutionary standpoint, ketones are the necessary alternative fuel.

The human species has evolved due to the ability to eat and digest the most unpredictable food. The survival of our ancestors depended on their ability to hunt and to find food all year round. Sometimes they didn't eat for a few days and even for several weeks if there was lack of plants and animals. People have evolved the ability to use and store various sources of fuel in order to be prepared for periodic food shortages. Conserved glycogen allowed to withstand the most part of the day without food, while stored fat provided a more stable source of fuel for longer periods of a lack of food.

Theoretically, the combination of glycogen and fat allows the human body to survive for weeks without food. In fact, there is one warning: The human brain requires a lot of energy for its work, and fatty acids cannot fully supply fuel to the brain cells. Fatty acids are processed too slowly, leaving the brain cells vulnerable to damage and starvation. That is why, in order to provide the brain with the required amount of energy, during the periods of fasting the liver converts non-sugar substrates, like amino acids, from protein into sugar through a process called gluconeogenesis. As a result of gluconeogenesis, the brain continues to function, but then it will have of muscle loss. We need to process up to 2.2 pounds of muscle mass in sugar every day in order to satisfy the energy needs of our brains during the famine. At this speed, the body will burn muscles too fast and won't have the strength to find food.

Fortunately, our bodies have developed the ability to produce ketones from the fat, as fuel, retaining muscle mass and providing energy to the brain during food shortages. Without ketosis, the body would be forced to use gluconeogenesis in order to stimulate the brain to burn the muscle mass.

Before you reach ketosis, your body will go through several stages:

Stage 1 - Glycogen exhaustion phase - from six to twenty-four hours from the moment the carbs intake was severely restricted or stopped

The level of insulin decreases, and glucagon level increases. Glucagon sends a signal to the liver that more sugar is needed in the blood. Thus, the liver destroys the accumulated glycogen in the muscles and increases gluconeogenesis.

Stage 2 - Gluconeogenic phase - from two to ten days of the carb restriction.

At this stage, glycogen runs almost completely low, and gluconeogenesis takes on the function of providing the body with energy. At the same time, the liver begins to produce acetoacetate, which can be turned into acetone. At this time, a person's breath can smell like a paint solvent. This phase lasts from two to ten days. Everything depends on your own glycogen deposits. It also depends on the level of the carbohydrates reduction. At this time, you can face a condition called a Keto flu. You may experience such symptoms as fatigue, headache, constipation, or diarrhea, as well as a great desire to eat anything sweet, flour, or starch. In general, the body requires carbohydrates as it used to consume. This period may be a reason for you to decide that the diet doesn't work. Another effect of the body's transition to ketosis, at a certain time, is an increasing of urination. Ketones are a natural diuretic, so you have to visit the WC often. Acetoacetate, a ketone body, is also excreted by urination, which is another factor affecting the frequency of urination. It is also a temporary phenomenon and passes after your body adapts to the new conditions. It is worth remembering that there is a conversion of your internal "power station" from coal to nuclear fuel, or from glucose to ketones. Please go easy on your body. If you do everything correctly, you may not even feel any of these symptoms. I had no side effects except the mild fatigue, but it lasted only a few days. I allowed myself to rest those days and kept physical activity to a minimum.

Stage 3 - Ketogenic phase - after seven to ten days of carb restriction

During this phase, the proteolysis reduces to generate energy, and the consumption of fats and ketones increases. At this time, your body goes into a state of ketosis. Everything is based on each person here. We are all different, and everyone enters this phase based upon his/her genetics, lifestyle factors, the level of activity, and a previous carb reduction.

Stage 4 - Keto-adaptation phase – from a few weeks to several months of carb reduction

After a couple of weeks, your body will be in a deep level of ketosis and will fully adapt to a new source of fuel. The requirement of glucose will decrease until the level that ketones can provide up to 50% of the body's energy needs.

These are four stages that you go through during the carb reduction or the limitation of food consuming in general. Your body will tell you when you are on the right track to ketosis.

Conclusion

All of these symptoms last no more than two weeks, but some of you may not feel them at all. However, if enough time has passed (more than ten days) and you still see some symptoms of transition, this may be a signal that your body cannot enter ketosis. If so, then you need to return to the beginning and revise your diet. Perhaps the amount of fat, proteins, and carbs is the wrong proportion. By reducing carbohydrates, you have imperceptibly increased the proteins. Be careful and keep them within twenty to twenty-five percent. Do not reduce the recommended amount of fat in food. Despite the fear of fat grounded on the long-standing eating habits, remember: Fat is your friend! Use it in the right proportion, and you will feel full and have lots of energy. As soon as you calculate and restart your diet, the unwell feeling will disappear, and you'll be able to enjoy all the benefits of ketosis!

If you want to know your level of ketosis, you can determine it by the number of ketones in your blood test.

Light ketosis: 0.5 mmol / L - 0.8 mmol / l

Average ketosis: 0.9 mmol / L - 1.4 mmol / l

Deep ketosis: 1.5 mmol / L - 3.0 mmol / l

Most of you will be in light ketosis for two or three days from the beginning of the ketogenic diet. Next, it will take from two to three weeks to enter the state of deep ketosis. Deep ketosis is ideal for weight loss and can bring some benefits as stabilization of psychological state, clarity of mind, and other things you could not get in an easy or medium ketosis. However, there is no need to fixate at the level of ketones in the blood. The most important thing is to follow the ketogenic diet properly, consuming the required food in the right proportion of macronutrients.

Who is this diet for?

When we consider the effects of ketosis, it becomes clear that it will help people with neurological problems most of all. When we trust our brain to ketones, we can reduce inflammation and damage of the neurons and improve the growth and functioning of the brain cells. The current studies of Alzheimer's and Parkinson's diseases, behavioral disorders of autism, and epilepsy indicate this statement is true.

Ketosis can also help fight such diseases as cancer, diabetes, and obesity. Ketones can improve the state of the body. This is due to the fact that ketones can help to reduce blood sugar levels and reduce appetite, which prevents us from consuming too many calories and too much sugar - the two main factors that cause such conditions as diabetes, obesity, and non-alcoholic fatty liver disease. It doesn't mean the diet helps only those people with the above-mentioned problems. Many healthy people can appreciate all advantages of ketosis. All you need is to reduce the carbs to the recommended minimum and follow the rules of a ketogenic diet. Some people note they feel an increase of cognitive function and a significant improvement of their health in general. However, the Keto diet has its disadvantages. Let us take a closer look at them.

Disadvantages of Keto

To adapt to the restriction of carbohydrates, the body experiences some significant changes. Not all of them are positive. For example, ketones increase the acid load on the body, which increases the protein requirements to help contain the pH balance with the additional nitrogen that amino acids provide. That's why it's important to make sure that you meet your protein requirements on a daily basis. If for some reason the acid buffer system of a person works incorrectly, which is rare, then ketosis can introduce your body into a state of acidosis.

Another important point, which you need to beware of, is the consumption of liquids and minerals. Because of the mild diuretic effect, you will be at a higher risk of mild dehydration and the symptoms of Keto flu while you are in ketosis. Make sure you drink a lot of water and minerals every day. Supporting the condition of ketosis causes problems for athletes. Anaerobic showings become worse using ketones and limiting glucose consumption. The effectiveness of endurance exercise, requiring intensive efforts, can be weakened by ketosis. Current research shows that ketosis reduces the effectiveness of high-intensity exercise - and it occurs regardless of the increase in ketones. On the other hand, ketosis improves or doesn't affect physical endurance with less intense muscles of the training process.

From my experience, I can say that, in addition to creatine and taurine, carbing in reasonable limits raises productivity rather than creatine and taurine.

Summary

Ketosis is a complex metabolic state that has many unique advantages. The healthiest way to achieve ketosis is to observe a ketogenic diet. In general, ketosis is safe and useful for most people. This is one of the main reasons why the ketogenic diet is so effective for improving health, well-being, and vitality raising. The complex of all these factors makes it so popular among people from different social classes and among housewives as well as film celebrities!

Attention, it is important!

Before you start, please consult a doctor who is competent in keto questions. Be sure to examine your liver and gallbladder and do all necessary tests. And if there are no obvious contraindications, then start your way to a new life bravely!

Starting the diet

To start a keto diet, you need to plan everything in advance. The first thing I advise is to find out your optimal weight, which complies with your age and sex. You can do it using free calculators, including keto calculators. They are available on the internet. After you figure out your optimal weight and the recommended caloric intake per day, based on your activity, you should make a week's menu. It's not difficult, knowing which products you can consume, the calorie content, and the percentage composition of the macronutrients. You can play in some kind of "constructor". It is good. There is a huge number of calculators for products and ready meals. As for me, it seemed complicated at first. Then, after three weeks on the diet, I found myself thinking about not counting calories anymore. My body became the best advisor.

When I started, my diet included eggs, bacon, beef, chicken, fatty cream, butter, mackerel, and almonds as well as a huge amount of broccoli, courgettes, and cabbage. I hated broccoli during my childhood, and now I have found these wonderful vegetables to be very good. I still caught myself thinking that there are too many greens in my diet than in keto. Therefore, I want to emphasize that it is important to listen to your body.

Now, if you haven't found any contraindications, tuned positively, and feel your strength develop, we will jump directly to the beginning of the diet.

Start to prepare your body gradually, refusing some products one by one. Slowly cut back on the number of carbohydrates, or just do it in one step dramatically reducing the intake of carbohydrates. Remember that our body is restructuring itself from one type of fuel to another, from sugar to fat. This stage can cause some difficulties. Previously your body extracted glucose from carbohydrates you consumed for dozens of years, and now, suddenly, the body is actually deprived of glucose. I can compare it with the feeling when somebody quits smoking. As mentioned earlier, you will have two ways to enter the diet.

The first method: You make an effort and limit the intake of carbs to twenty to thirty grams daily. Do it for one day.

The second method: You gradually cut back on the intake of carbs for seven to ten days, but no more. For example, you set a bar of carbohydrate intake in the range of 100 - 130 grams, and then remove ten grams every day. Your body will react calmer on cutting back on carbs with this method.

It is your personal choice on how to enter ketosis. But the right thing is to listen to your body. Looking back at my experience, I can say I did it as well as I quit smoking. I refused all carbs at once without stretching this "pleasure" for a week. The good news is that it's pretty easy to maintain the low carbs intake from the first days, thanks to the food that really nourish! But then again, it all depends on the individual characteristics of the body and the ability of your metabolism to adapt itself quickly.

The next step is to control the stock in your fridge and pantry in order to cut out some products and replace them with the products in the keto diet.

You need to cut out the following

Sugar: first and foremost, sweets, sweet drinks, fruit juices, energetics, white and chocolate milk, any pastry, confectionery, ice cream, cereals, muesli. If you have a dependency and a painful craving for sweets, you should avoid even sweeteners for some time.

Starch: bread, pastries, pasta, potatoes, chips and snacks, whole grains, almost all cereals, and cereals (except for chickpeas, flax, and sesame, but in small quantities). You can eat roots like carrots but in small amounts and with a minimum of heat treatment.

Margarine and most vegetable oils. The reason is the presence of harmful trans fats and omega-6 acids of a questionable utility in composition.

Beer, tinctures, and sweet liqueurs.

Fruits and dried fruits: fruits contain a lot of sugar and fructose so try to use them rarely, except avocado and coconut.

Allowed food for you

Meat: any for your taste. Veal, pork, lamb, poultry, etc. Don't throw away pieces of fat from meat and poultry skin. If possible, it is better to choose the farm meat of animals, which were fed in a traditional way

Fish and seafood: any, but the best option is fatty fish such as salmon, salmon mackerel, and herring. Also, prawns and squid are welcome.

Eggs: in any form.

Seasonal vegetables: all kinds of lettuce, cabbage, zucchini, asparagus, olives, spinach, cucumbers, tomatoes, peppers, spring onions, any greens, pumpkin, etc. In general, there is a simple rule: eat food that grows above ground, and try not to eat food that grows underground.

Mushrooms: any edible.

Dairy products: fat cream (twenty to forty percent), fatty sour cream, cottage cheese, Greek yogurt, fatty cheeses. Be careful with sour-milk, flavored foods with additives and **low-fat content** - basically, they contain a lot of sugar, thickeners, and other dubious ingredients. The best way is to buy sour-milk products on farms that you trust or to cook it at home from milk and dry sourdough.

Nuts and seeds: macadamia, walnuts, almonds, sunflower seeds, and pumpkins.

Berries: in small quantities, in case you don't maintain a strict regime in terms of carbs. Raspberries, blackberries, and other berries with a low glycemic index are suitable.

Allowed drinks

Pure water.

Drip coffee, especially with cream.

Tea and herbal decoctions to your taste.

Drinks and products are allowed sometimes

Alcohol: dry wines, not sweet strong drinks (gin, rum, whiskey, vodka), not sweet cocktails.

Black chocolate: in very moderate quantities, with a cocoa content of more than eighty-five percent.

Fats and oils

Fats will make up most of your daily calorie consumption when you are on a ketogenic diet, so the choice should be made in consideration of your likes and dislikes. They can be combined in different ways, giving you different flavours to your dishes.

Fats are vital to our body, but they can also be dangerous if you consume the wrong types of fats. There are several different kinds of fats that are involved in a ketogenic diet. Different foods usually contain diverse combinations of fats, but unhealthy fats should be avoided. Here is a brief overview:

Saturated fats. You can eat: butter, melted butter, coconut oil, lard, and MST oil.

Monounsaturated fats. You can eat: olive oil, avocado oil, and macadamia.

Polyunsaturated fats. You have to know the difference. You can find polyunsaturated fats in animal protein and oily fish are great for you, and you should eat them. Processed polyunsaturated fats are harmful for you.

Trans fats. You have to avoid trans fats completely. These are processed fats that are chemically altered (hydrogenated) to improve expire date. Please avoid all hydrogenated fats, such as margarine, because consumption of such kind of fats is one of the factors leading to the heart diseases

Some keto recipes involve the usage of rare products such as Golden Flaxseed Meal, Chia Seeds, Liquid Stevia, MCT100% Oil, Xanthan Gum, almond flour, erythritol, psyllium husk powder and so on, which are not sold at regular stores. You can find them on Amazon.

There is one small nuance. You are on your way to the keto-friendly products. If you live alone, or with a person who fully supports you and is ready to do this with you, then it will be simple to clean out your fridge and pantry. But what will you do if you live in a big family, the food preferences and traditions of which were formed during the dozens of years and were inherited after previous generations? Well, do you have to buy another fridge or to construct one more pantry for yourself? Of course, no! You can find some space in your fridge to place the products for your diet.

It is clear your new way of eating will cause a lot of questions from your relatives. They may even make fun of you at the beginning. But you'll need to have patience and ignore them! Or am I exaggerating too much? Well, all families are different. Let's hope you will have support and understanding. In any case, as soon as you make good progress, some of the critical voices will want to follow the Keto diet, too! And it is possible that you will become the reformer who will lead your family to a new life, full of health and energy!

So, you're ready!

Your health has no contraindication, and your mood is the most positive! The necessary products are stored in the fridge and pantry. Some of you are lucky to have relatives who believe in you and some of you have no support team.

There are some edifications before you start:

1) *Keep a diary of consumed food* or install the appropriate application on your smartphone. It will allow you to be more responsible while eating. Write down everything, including small snacks. At the end of the day, you will see the whole picture. Many of you will be surprised with the amount of food eaten, but it will give you a chance to correct your diet in case you need to do so.

2) *Find somebody you can trust* who will record all your achievements and hold you accountable. Many people become more organized when they have to report to someone. So it will give you an additional sense of responsibility. Sometimes he/she will praise and encourage you, which is very important in the beginning and gives you extra strength!

3) *Drink plenty of water*. This is an important reminder. It is difficult to overestimate the value of water in ketosis. Your body needs more water to burn fat than for burning glucose.

4) *Do not overdo the sweeteners*, Artificial sweeteners are the same refined food as sugar. The main difference is that they do not have an immediate effect on blood sugar. You need to know the measure because uncontrolled consumption of sweeteners increases the obsession with usual sugar!

5) *Try to avoid stressful situations and control your emotions*. Stress increases the level of cortisol, which, in turn, increases the level of sugar. This can provoke a desire to eat something sweet.

6) *When you go to bed too late*, cortisol is produced in great quantities. That's why you feel hungry when your sleep mode is broken. Keep a check on it. Remember, a timely sleep is a guarantee of a chipper mood!

7) *Do not be distracted* by anything else during your meal! It keeps you from eating too much. If you concentrate on the food itself during a meal, the feeling of nourishment comes quickly, and the probability of eating an extra piece goes away.

8) *As for physical activity*, I don't encourage you to go to the nearest sports club and exercise until you are blue in the face. Of course, not! But please, include some biking, running, swimming, walking, or some kind of exercising. The diet and some physical activity will give you excellent results! Your goal is not just to lose weight but also to keep the muscles toned. As a bonus, you will receive "many thanks" from the cardiovascular and central nervous systems, improving the general condition of the body and changing your mood, for sure!

In the next chapters, you'll find the recipes

You can create your own menu depending on your preferences. By now you have already calculated the required number of calories per day. Based on this calculation you can choose the dishes and adjust the portions to your needs.

14 Day Meal Plan

Here you are presented with two-week food plan with three meals consisting of 1500-1700 cal / per day. It's a base. You can easily regulate the calorie and fat content of your daily ration with an additional snack, a handful of nuts, for example. You can also add an extra spoon of butter / cream to the dish.

The nutrition plan contains repeating recipes. This was made for your convenience, so you can save your time and cook several portions for a couple of days. The main goal you need to achieve in these two weeks is to start the process of ketosis. After the adaptation process is over and you get used to the new state, you can choose any of the presented recipes. You will make a menu according to your abilities and preferences. Hereafter, knowing the principles of the keto diet, you can easily think up the dishes from the right products, without calculating of calories, only listening for your body!

I would be sincerely happy if my example and experience help you to attain the goals you have set!

Sincerely yours, Adam

Week 1

Day 1

Breakfast   Crustless Quiches…………………………………………………………….32

Lunch   Cheddar and Ham Wraps……………………………………………….162

Dinner   Tasty Chicken with Mushrooms……………………………………...74

Total calories – *1611 Fat – 121.4g Carbs – 18.3g Protein – 94.1g*

Day 2

Breakfast   Crustless Quiches…………………………………………………………….32

Lunch   Easy Avocado Wraps…………………………………………………….163

Dinner   Low Carb Chicken Quesadilla……………………………………….69

Total calories – *1661 Fat – 126.2g Carbs – 18.3g Protein – 91.1g*

Day 3

Breakfast   Crustless Quiches…………………………………………………………….32

Lunch   Cobb Salad…………………………………………………………………….128

Dinner   Cheddar Chicken and Broccoli Casserole……………………….72

Total calories – *1518 Fat – 113.4g Carbs – 11.4g Protein – 107.3g*

Day 4

Breakfast Delicious Chocolate Peanut Butter Muffins..189

Lunch   Avocado Tuna Salad...94

Dinner   Cheddar Chicken and Broccoli Casserole...72

Total calories – *1588 Fat – 116.3g Carbs – 13.4g Protein – 88.3g*

Day 5

Breakfast Delicious Chocolate Peanut Butter Muffins..189

Lunch   Cheddar Chicken and Broccoli Casserole...72

Dinner   Shrimp and Mushroom Zucchini Pasta..102

Total calories – *1573 Fat – 114.4g Carbs – 15.7g Protein – 102g*

Day 6

Breakfast Delicious Chocolate Peanut Butter Muffins..189

Lunch   Cheddar Chicken and Broccoli Casserole...72

Dinner   Sriracha Lime Flank Steak..87

Total calories – *1631 Fat – 117.6g Carbs – 16.2g Protein – 111.5g*

Day 7

Breakfast Creamy Scrambled Eggs..41

Lunch   Chicken Zucchini Noodles Soup...78

Dinner   Low Carb Bunless Butter Burger...93

Total calories – *1698 Fat – 143.5g Carbs – 11.6g Protein – 104.9 g*

Week 2

Day 1

Total calories – *1437 Fat – 106g Carbs – 15.85g Protein – 99.2g*

Day 2

Total calories – *1646 Fat – 122.5g Carbs – 16.55g Protein – 115.8g*

Day 3

Total calories – *1455 Fat – 112.3g Carbs – 16.2g Protein – 99.3g*

Day 4

Total calories – 1712 Fat – 127.3g Carbs – 13.45 Protein – 133.6g

Day 5

Total calories – 1511 Fat – 108.5g Carbs – 16.7g Protein – 93.3g

Day 6

Total calories – 1544 Fat – 106.2g Carbs – 12.9g Protein – 120.6g

Day 7

Total calories – 1547 Fat – 124.8g Carbs – 11g Protein – 121.2 g

Eggs and Sausages

Prep time: 15 minutes | Cook time: 40 minutes | Servings: 6

Ingredients:

2 sausages

1 onion, medium

5 tbsp butter

1 red bell pepper

Salt and ground black pepper to taste

12 ham slices

1 oz spinach, torn

12 eggs

Directions:

1. Chop onion and sausages.
2. Preheat pan over medium heat. Add 1 tablespoon of butter, add onion and sausages. Cook for 5 minutes, stirring occasionally.
3. Scoop out seeds and chop bell pepper.
4. Add bell pepper, salt and ground black pepper to pan, mix well and cook for 3 minutes.
5. Transfer mixture to bowl.
6. Add 4 tablespoons butter to pan and melt it. Divide butter into 12 ramekins.
7. Add slice of ham to each ramekin.
8. Divide spinach and sausage mixture in each ramekin
9. Preheat oven to 425 F.
10. Crack egg on top of each ramekin, place in oven and bake for 20 minutes.
11. Let cool for 5-10 minutes and serve.

Nutrition per Serving: Calories - 438, Carbs – 11.8, Fat – 31.5g, Protein – 21.8g

Sausage and Broccoli Quiche

Prep time: 20 minutes | Cook time: 60 minutes | Servings: 8

Ingredients:

½ lb breakfast sausage

1 cup broccoli

2 cups almond flour

1 tbsp sea salt

2 tbsp coconut oil

9 eggs

2 tbsp water

Directions:

1. Cook the sausage and set aside.
2. Divide broccoli into florets. Steam and set aside.
3. Using food processor, blend almond flour and sea salt.
4. Add coconut oil and 1 egg and continue blending to form a ball.
5. Pour dough into a quiche pan. Top with sausage and broccoli.
6. In another bowl, whisk together 8 eggs and water.
7. Pour mixture over sausage and broccoli.
8. Preheat oven to 350 F.
9. Place dish in oven and bake for 35 minutes.
10. Serve.

Nutrition per Serving: Calories – 340, Carbs - 6g, Fat – 23.8g, Protein - 17.8g

Crustless Quiches

Prep time: 20 minutes | Cook time: 30 minutes | Servings: 3

Ingredients:

14 medium eggs, beaten

1/3 cup heavy cream

1 tsp kosher salt

2/3 cup mozzarella cheese

1 tbsp olive oil

3 plum tomatoes, chopped

1/3 cup sweet Vidalia onion

1 tsp ground black pepper

2/3 cup soppressata salami

1/3 cup sliced pickled jalapenos

1/3 cup pepper jack

½ tsp cayenne

Directions:

1. Set oven to 325 F and heat it up.
2. Grease 11" to 15" cupcake tin.
3. In big bowl, whisk together eggs, heavy cream and salt.
4. Add mozzarella cheese, olive oil, tomatoes, sweet Vidalia onion, black pepper, salami, jalapenos, cayenne, and pepper jack. Stir well.
5. Spread batter in cupcake tin and place in oven. Bake for 25 minutes.
6. Serve warm.

Nutrition per 4 Crustless Quiches: Calories - 379, Carbs – 5.5, Fat – 27.9g, Protein – 21.8g

Cauliflower Fritters

Prep time: 15 minutes | Cook time: 12 minutes | Servings: 6

Ingredients:

1½ lbs cauliflower, washed and chopped

1 oz almond flour

1 tsp salt

1 tsp paprika

1 tbsp mustard

1 tsp basil

¼ tsp red chili pepper

3 cloves garlic, peeled and minced

2 tbsp almond milk

1 large egg, beaten

7 oz ground chicken

1 tbsp olive oil

Directions:

1. Place cauliflower in food processor and blend it until the texture is smooth.
2. Transfer mixture to bowl and add almond flour, salt, paprika, mustard, and basil.
3. Stir it to reach homogeneous texture.
4. Add red chili pepper, garlic and almond milk.
5. Add egg and stir just until combined and texture of fritter dough is smooth.
6. Add chicken and mix well.
7. Heat up non-stick pan and pour olive oil.
8. Shape fritters and place them on preheated pan.
9. Cook fritters for 3 minutes on both sides.
10. After Cook fritters place them on paper towel to remove excess oil.
11. Serve warm.

Nutrition per Serving: Calories - 178, Carbs – 8.9g, Fat – 9.9g, Protein - 14.9g

Broccoli and Cheddar Biscuits

Prep time: 15 minutes | Cook time: 30 minutes | Servings: 12

Ingredients:

1½ cups almond flour

½ tsp baking soda

1 tsp paprika

1 tsp garlic powder

Salt and ground black pepper to taste

¼ cup coconut oil

2 eggs, beaten

½ tsp apple cider vinegar

2 cups cheddar cheese, grated

4 cups broccoli florets

Directions:

1. In medium bowl, mix together almond flour, baking soda, paprika, garlic powder, salt and pepper to taste.
2. Stir in coconut oil, vinegar, eggs and cheddar cheese.
3. Place broccoli florets, salt and pepper to taste in blender or food processor and blend well.
4. Add broccoli mixture to bowl and mix well.
5. Preheat oven to 375 F.
6. Shape 12 patties and place on baking sheet. Cook for 20 minutes.
7. Then place under broiler for 5 minutes.
8. Serve hot.

Nutrition per Serving: Calories - 165, Carbs – 2g, Fat – 12.5g, Protein – 7.2g

Corndogs

Prep time: 15 minutes | Cook time: 12 minutes | Servings: 4

Ingredients:

1 tsp baking powder

¼ tsp cayenne pepper

1 cup almond meal

½ tsp turmeric

1 tsp Italian seasoning

Salt and ground black pepper to taste

2 tbsp heavy cream

2 eggs

4 sausages

1½ cups olive oil

Directions:

1. In a medium bowl, mix together baking powder, cayenne pepper, almond meal, turmeric, Italian seasoning, salt and pepper. Set aside.
2. In another bowl, whisk together heavy cream and eggs.
3. Pour egg mixture into almond meal mixture and stir to combine.
4. Toss sausages in bowl until they are covered in mixture.
5. Pour oil in pan and preheat over medium-high heat.
6. Transfer sausages to pan and cook for 2 minutes per side.
7. Place cooked sausages on plate, drain grease and serve.

Nutrition per Serving: Calories - 340, Carbs – 5.2g, Fat – 32g, Protein – 16.7g

Shrimp and Bacon Breakfast

Prep time: 15 minutes | Cook time: 17 minutes | Servings: 4

Ingredients:

1 cup mushrooms

4 bacon slices

4 oz smoked salmon, chopped

4 oz shrimp, deveined

Salt and ground black pepper to taste

½ cup coconut cream

Directions:

1. Preheat pan over medium heat.
2. Meanwhile, chop bacon. Add bacon to pan and cook for 5 minutes.
3. Slice mushrooms and add to pan, cook for another 5 minutes, stirring occasionally.
4. Add salmon and stir. Cook for 3 minutes more.
5. Add shrimp and stir. Cook for 2 minutes more.
6. Sprinkle with salt and pepper, stir.
7. Add coconut cream, stir and cook for another 1 minute.
8. Serve warm.

Nutrition per Serving: Calories - 335, Carbs – 4.2g, Fat – 24g, Protein – 17.5g

Delicious Keto Yogurt

Prep time: 10 minutes| Cook time: 12 minutes | Servings: 5

Ingredients:

1 oz cream

¼ cup cream cheese

2 cups almond milk

2 tbsp Erythritol

2 oz hazelnuts, crushed

½ cup raspberries, sliced

Directions:

1. Place cream and cream cheese in blender or food processor and blend until texture is smooth.
2. Pour in almond milk and blend mixture for another 1 minute.
3. Transfer cream mixture to a bowl and add Erythritol.
4. Add crushed hazelnuts and mix carefully.
5. Sprinkle yogurt with raspberries.
6. Serve immediately or store in fridge.

Nutrition per Serving: Calories – 349, Carbs - 11.9g, Fat - 34.9g, Protein - 4.9g

Pizza Dip

Prep time: 15 minutes | Cook time: 22 minutes | Servings: 4

Ingredients:

¼ cup sour cream

½ cup mozzarella cheese

4 oz cream cheese, softened

¼ cup mayonnaise

Salt and ground black pepper to taste

½ cup tomato sauce

¼ cup Parmesan cheese, grated

1 tbsp green bell pepper, seeded and chopped

6 pepperoni slices, chopped

½ tsp Italian seasoning

4 black olives, pitted and chopped

Directions:

1. In medium bowl, mix together sour cream, mozzarella cheese, cream cheese, mayonnaise, salt and pepper.
2. Put mixture into 4 ramekins.
3. Add in such orders: layer of tomato sauce, layer Parmesan cheese, chopped bell peppers, chopped pepperoni, Italian seasoning, chopped black olives.
4. Preheat oven to 350 F.
5. Place ramekins in oven and cook for 20 minutes. Serve.

Nutrition per Serving: Calories - 399, Carbs – 3.9g, Fat – 33.7g, Protein – 14.9g

Mexican Breakfast

Prep time: 15 minutes | Cook time: 32 minutes | Servings: 8

Ingredients:

1 lb chorizo

1 lb ground pork

½ cup enchilada sauce

8 medium eggs

3 tbsp butter

Salt and ground black pepper to taste

4 oz onion, chopped

1 tomato, cored and chopped

1 avocado, pitted, peeled, and chopped

Directions:

1. Chop chorizo and mix well with ground pork.
2. Transfer mixture to baking sheet.
3. Top with enchilada sauce.
4. Preheat oven to 350 F.
5. Place baking sheet in oven and cook for 20 minutes.
6. In bowl, whisk eggs with salt and pepper.
7. Preheat pan over medium heat and melt butter.
8. Pour egg mixture in pan and cook slowly until eggs set, stirring now and then.
9. When pork mixture is cooked, place scrambled eggs over it.
10. Sprinkle with salt and pepper.
11. Top with onion, tomato and avocado. Serve.

Nutrition per Serving: Calories - 398, Carbs – 6.8g, Fat – 33g, Protein – 24.8g

Feta Omelet

Prep time: 12 minutes | Cook time: 11 minutes | Servings: 1

Ingredients:

1 tbsp heavy cream

3 eggs, beaten

Salt and ground black pepper to taste

1 tbsp butter

1 oz feta cheese, crumbled

1 tbsp jarred pesto

Directions:

1. Whisk together heavy cream, eggs, salt and pepper.
2. Preheat pan over medium high heat and melt butter.
3. Pour in egg mixture and cook omelet until it's fluffy.
4. Sprinkle with cheese and pesto.
5. Fold omelet in half and cover pan. Cook for 5 minutes more.
6. Serve.

Nutrition per Serving: Calories - 497, Carbs – 3.1g, Fat – 44g, Protein – 29.5g

Creamy Scrambled Eggs

Prep time: 10 minutes | Cook time: 7 minutes | Servings: 1

Ingredients:

2 tbsp butter

4 large eggs, beaten

2 tbsp sour cream

½ tsp salt

¼ tsp black pepper

4 strips bacon

1 stalk green onion, chopped

Directions:

1. Preheat pan on medium heat and melt butter.
2. Add eggs and cook, stirring constantly.
3. When eggs are almost done, add sour cream and cook for 30 seconds more.
4. Sprinkle with salt and pepper and transfer to plate.
5. Add bacon strips to pan and let them cook for 1 minute on both sides.
6. Top eggs and bacons with green onion and serve.

Nutrition per Serving: Calories – 695, Carbs – 2.65g, Fat – 58g, Protein – 58.2g

Morning Pie

Prep time: 15 minutes | Cook time: 18 minutes | Servings: 4

Ingredients:

3 oz Parmesan cheese, sliced into thick pieces

5 medium eggs, beaten

8 oz full-fat cream cheese

4 cloves garlic, peeled and minced

1 tsp salt

½ tsp cayenne pepper

1 tbsp butter

4 oz cream

Directions:

1. Put Parmesan cheese in baking form.
2. Place baking form in oven and cook for about 5 minutes on 360 F.
3. In medium bowl, whisk eggs. Add cream cheese and mix well.
4. In another bowl, combine garlic with salt and cayenne pepper.
5. Add garlic to egg mixture and stir well.
6. Heat up a pan, add and melt butter.
7. Pour egg mixture in pan and cook for 3 minutes on medium high heat, stirring constantly.
8. Place scrambled eggs on Parmesan cheese in baking form.
9. Top with cream and back baking form to oven. Cook for 10 minutes on 360 F.
10. Remove dish from oven and let it cool for about 10 minutes. Serve.

Nutrition per Serving: Calories - 389, Carbs – 4.9g, Fat - 34.7g, Protein - 18g

Blender Pancakes

Prep time: 10 minutes | Cook time: 12 minutes | Servings: 1

Ingredients:

2 large eggs, beaten

1 scoop vanilla protein powder

2 oz cream cheese

10 drops liquid stevia

¼ tsp salt

1/8 tsp cinnamon

Directions:

1. Place eggs, vanilla and cream cheese in blender or food processor and pulse it well.
2. Add liquid stevia, salt and cinnamon to food processor and blend until smooth.
3. Preheat pan on medium heat and spread pancake batter into 4-5" diameter rounds.
4. Bake on both sides until cooked.
5. Serve with sugar free maple syrup or butter.

Nutrition per Serving: Calories – 445, Carbs – 3.9g, Fat – 28.5g, Protein – 40.6g

Sausage Patties

Prep time: 15 minutes | Cook time: 12 minutes | Servings: 4

Ingredients:

1 lb minced pork

Salt and ground black pepper to taste

½ tsp sage, dried

¼ tsp thyme, dried

¼ tsp ground ginger

3 tbsp cold water

1 tbsp coconut oil

Directions:

1. In small bowl, combine salt, sage, pepper, thyme, ginger and water.
2. In medium bowl, combine spice mix with pork.
3. Make patties and set aside.
4. Add coconut oil to pan and preheat it on medium high heat.
5. Transfer patties to pan and cook for 5 minutes, then flip, and cook them for 3 minutes more.
6. Serve.

Nutrition per Serving: Calories - 318, Carbs – 11g, Fat – 12.8g, Protein – 11.8g

Keto Breakfast Mix

Prep time: 20 minutes | Cook time: 22 minutes | Servings: 6

Ingredients:

1 tsp turmeric

½ tsp oregano

1 tsp cilantro

1 tsp salt

½ tsp ground black pepper

1 tsp paprika

1¼ cup bacon, chopped

1 tbsp butter

5.5 oz white mushrooms, sliced

1¼ cup zucchini, diced

5.5 oz cauliflower, divided into florets

5.5 oz asparagus, cut in half

2 cloves garlic

1 white onion, sliced

1 cup chicken broth

Directions:

1. In small bowl, mix together turmeric, oregano, cilantro, salt, pepper, and paprika.
2. Season bacon with spice mixture, stir well.
3. Heat up a pan, add and melt butter.
4. Add bacon to pan and cook for 5 minutes on medium heat, stirring constantly.
5. Add mushrooms, zucchini and cauliflower, stir and cook for another 2 minutes.
6. Stir in asparagus, garlic and onion and pour chicken broth.
7. Simmer for 10 minutes until vegetables are softened.
8. Serve warm.

Nutrition per Serving: Calories - 308, Carbs - 8.3g, Fat - 21.9g, Protein - 21g

Sausage Quiche

Prep time: 15 minutes | Cook time: 45 minutes | Servings: 6

Ingredients:

12 oz pork sausage

5 eggplants

10 mixed cherry tomatoes, halved

6 eggs, beaten

2 tsp whipping cream

2 tbsp Parmesan cheese, grated

2 tbsp fresh parsley, chopped

Salt and ground black pepper to taste

Directions:

1. Chop sausage and place on the bottom of a baking dish.
2. Slice eggplants and lay on top.
3. Lay cherry tomatoes on eggplant.
4. In a medium bowl, combine eggs, cream, Parmesan cheese, parsley, salt and pepper.
5. Pour mixture over tomatoes.
6. Preheat oven to 375 F.
7. Place baking dish in oven and cook for 40 minutes.
8. Top with parsley and serve.

Nutrition per Serving: Calories - 338, Carbs – 2.9g, Fat – 27.5g, Protein – 17.1g

Sausage with Egg and Cheese

Prep time: 10 minutes | Cook time: 7 minutes | Servings: 1

Ingredients:

1 tsp olive oil

1 large egg, beaten

3 oz breakfast sausage, cooked

1 slice cheddar cheese

Green onion, chopped (for garnish)

Directions:

1. Heat up pan with olive oil over medium heat, add eggs and fry until cooked (sunny side up or over easy).
2. Transfer to plate with cooked sausage and cheddar cheese.
3. Sprinkle with green onion and serve with your favorite hot sauce.

Nutrition per Serving: Calories – 404, Carbs – 1.1g, Fat – 42g, Protein – 26g

Eggplant Stew

Prep time: 15 minutes | Cook time: 25 minutes | Servings: 6

Ingredients:

1 zucchini, sliced

1 cup chorizo sausages, sliced

½ tsp cayenne pepper

1 tsp basil

2 cups chicken broth

1 white onion, peeled and diced

1 cup eggplants, peeled and chopped

1 tbsp coconut oil

1 tsp salt

Directions:

1. In bowl, mix together zucchini and sausages.
2. Season with cayenne pepper and basil. Stir well.
3. Heat up pan and add chicken broth.
4. Add zucchini with sausages, onion, eggplant, and coconut oil.
5. Sprinkle with salt and stir.
6. Close lid and simmer dish for 20-25 minutes on medium heat.
7. After Cook stir carefully and serve.

Nutrition per Serving: Calories - 234, Carbs - 7g, Fat – 17.8g, Protein – 10.8g

Chicken Omelet

Prep time: 15 minutes | Cook time: 15 minutes | Servings: 1

Ingredients:

2 eggs, beaten

Salt and ground black pepper to taste

Olive oil spray

1 oz rotisserie chicken, cooked and shredded

1 tomato, cored and chopped

2 bacon slices, crumbled

1 small avocado, peeled and chopped

1 tbsp mayonnaise

1 tsp mustard

Directions:

1. In medium bowl, whisk together eggs, salt and pepper.
2. Preheat the pan on medium heat, add some Cook oil, pour in egg mixture and cook for 5 minutes.
3. Place chicken, tomato, bacon, avocado, mayonnaise and mustard on one half of omelet. Then fold omelet.
4. Close pan with lid and cook for about 5 minutes.
5. Serve warm.

Nutrition per Serving: Calories - 400, Carbs – 3.8, Fat – 31g, Protein – 26

Pepperoni Pizza Omelet

Prep time: 15 minutes | Cook time: 12 minutes | Servings: 1

Ingredients:

Cooking spray

3 large eggs, beaten

1 tbsp heavy cream

4 oz pepperoni slices

4 oz mozzarella cheese, shredded

Salt and ground black pepper to taste

Dried basil to taste

2 bacon strips

Directions:

1. Preheat pan on medium heat and drizzle with cooking spray.
2. In bowl, combine eggs with heavy cream.
3. Pour mixture in pan and cook until almost done. Then add some pepperoni slices to one side.
4. Sprinkle cheese, black pepper, salt and basil over pepperoni and fold omelet over.
5. Cook for 1 minute more.
6. Meanwhile, in another pan fry bacon strips until cooked.
7. Serve omelet with cooked bacon.

Nutrition per Serving: Calories – 591, Carbs – 4.9g, Fat – 54g, Protein – 31.7g

Kale Fritters

Prep time: 15 minutes | Cook time: 10 minutes | Servings: 6

Ingredients:

7 oz kale, chopped (tiny pieces)

10 oz zucchini, washed and grated

1 tsp basil

½ tsp salt

¼ cup almond flour

½ tbsp mustard

1 large egg

1 tbsp coconut milk

1 white onion, diced

1 tbsp olive oil

Directions:

1. In medium bowl, mix together kale and zucchini.
2. Add basil and salt and stir.
3. Add almond flour and mustard. Stir well.
4. In another bowl, whisk together egg, coconut milk and onion.
5. Pour egg mixture into zucchini mixture and knead thick dough.
6. Preheat pan with olive oil on medium heat.
7. Shape fritters with help of spoon and put them in pan.
8. Cook fritters for about 2 minutes per side.
9. Transfer fritters to paper towel to remove excess oil.
10. Serve hot.

Nutrition per Serving: Calories - 120, Carbs – 8.8g, Fat – 8g, Protein - 5g

Italian Spaghetti Casserole

Prep time: 15 minutes | Cook time: 50 minutes | Servings: 6

Ingredients:

1 spaghetti squash, halved

Salt and ground black pepper to taste

4 tbsp butter

2 cloves garlic

1 cup onion

4 oz tomatoes

3 oz Italian salami, chopped

½ cup Kalamata olives, chopped

½ tsp Italian seasoning

4 medium eggs

½ cup fresh parsley, chopped

Directions:

1. Heat up oven to 400 F.
2. Put squash on baking sheet. Sprinkle with salt and pepper.
3. Add 1 tablespoon butter and place in oven. Cook for 45 minutes.
4. Meanwhile, peel and mince garlic; peel and chop onion; core and chop tomatoes.
5. Preheat pan on medium heat, add and melt 3 tablespoons butter.
6. Add onion, garlic, salt and pepper, sauté for 2 minutes, stirring occasionally.
7. Add chopped tomatoes and chopped salami. Stir and cook for 10 minutes.
8. Add chopped olives and Italian seasoning. Stir and cook for 2-3 minutes more.
9. Remove squash halves from oven and scrape flesh with fork.
10. Combine spaghetti squash with salami mixture in pan.
11. Shape 4 spaces in mixture and crack egg in each.
12. Sprinkle with salt and pepper and place pan in oven.
13. Cook at 400 F until eggs are done.
14. Top with parsley and serve.

Nutrition per Serving: Calories - 328, Carbs – 11.9, Fat – 24g, Protein – 16

Cream Cheese Soufflé

Prep time: 15 minutes | Cook time: 20 minutes | Servings: 4

Ingredients:

1/3 cup spinach, chopped roughly

1 tsp coconut oil

¼ cup white onion, peeled and diced

1 egg, beaten

½ cup cream cheese

¼ cup coconut flour

1 tsp salt

1 tsp paprika

Directions:

1. Place spinach in blender or food processor and blend until texture smooth.
2. Preheat pan with coconut oil on medium heat.
3. Add onion and sauté for about 5 minutes, stirring constantly, until onion turn golden brown.
4. In medium bowl, combine egg, cream cheese and coconut flour.
5. Season mixture with salt and paprika, stir well.
6. Add cooked onion to mixture and stir.
7. Pour soufflé in baking dish.
8. Place dish in oven at 365 F and bake for 10 minutes
9. Remove baking dish from oven and whisk it carefully. Serve.

Nutrition per Serving: Calories - 196, Carbs - 5.3g, Fat – 16.9g, Protein - 5.6g

Morning Casserole

Prep time: 20 minutes | Cook time: 25 minutes | Servings: 4

Ingredients:

3 eggs, beaten

8 oz ground chicken

1 tsp salt

1 tsp oregano

½ tsp dried basil

1 tsp dried cilantro

½ tsp cayenne pepper

2 green bell peppers, deseeded and chopped

1 and 1/3 cup cauliflower, divided into florets

1 tbsp olive oil

6 oz Cheddar cheese, grated

Directions:

1. In medium bowl, combine eggs with chicken.
2. Season mixture with salt, oregano, basil, cilantro and cayenne pepper. Stir well.
3. In another bowl, mix together bell peppers and cauliflower.
4. Grease baking dish with olive oil.
5. Add chicken mixture to baking dish, lay cauliflower mixture on top, and sprinkle with Cheddar cheese.
6. Cover baking dish tightly with aluminum foil.
7. Place form in oven at 360F and cook for 10 minutes.
8. Remove foil and bake dish for another 10 minutes.
9. Remove baking dish from oven and let it cook for 5-7 minutes. Serve.

Nutrition per Serving: Calories - 229, Carbs - 5.4g, Fat - 16g, Protein - 17.8g

Breakfast Bread

Prep time: 12 minutes | Cook time: 5 minutes | Servings: 4

Ingredients:

1 egg, beaten

⅓ cup almond flour

2½ tbsp coconut oil

½ tsp baking powder

A pinch of salt

Directions:

1. Whisk together egg, almond flour, oil, baking powder and salt.
2. Grease a microwave-safe form with some coconut oil.
3. Pour egg mixture into form and place in microwave.
4. Cook for 3 minutes on high heat.
5. When bread is cooked, let it cool for 5-10 minutes.
6. Slice and serve.

Nutrition per Serving: Calories - 119, Carbs – 2.8g, Fat – 11.8g, Protein – 4.2g

Naan Bread

Prep time: 15 minutes | Cook time: 15 minutes | Servings: 4

Ingredients:

½ cup coconut flour

½ tsp baking powder

1/3 tsp salt

1 cup water

1 tbsp coconut oil

3 tbsp butter

1 tbsp garlic, minced

Directions:

1. In medium bowl, mix together coconut flour, baking powder, salt and water.
2. Mix mass until dough is smooth and elastic.
3. Shape balls from dough and flatten them.
4. Grease pan with oil and heat it up on medium heat.
5. Transfer balls to pan and cook naan bread for about 5 minutes on both sides, until you get golden color.
6. In small sauté pan, melt butter and combine with garlic. Stir well.
7. Pour garlic mixture over bread and serve hot.

Nutrition per Serving: Calories - 130, Carbs – 2.9g, Fat – 12.9g, Protein - 0.8g

Pesto Crackers

Prep time: 15 minutes | Cook time: 20 minutes | Servings: 4

Ingredients:

1 clove garlic

1¼ cups almond flour

Salt and ground black pepper to taste

½ tsp baking powder

¼ tsp dried basil

A pinch of cayenne pepper

2 tbsp basil pesto

3 tbsp butter, softened

Directions:

1. Peel and mince garlic.
2. Combine almond flour, pepper, salt and baking powder.
3. Add dried basil, cayenne pepper, minced garlic and pesto. Mix well.
4. Add butter and stir dough with your hand.
5. Preheat oven to 325 F.
6. Pour dough on baking sheet and place in oven. Cook for 17 minutes.
7. Let it cool for 20-30 minutes, cut and serve.

Nutrition per Serving: Calories - 198, Carbs – 3.9, Fat - 19, Protein – 6.8

Jalapeño Balls

Prep time: 15 minutes | Cook time: 15 minutes | Servings: 3

Ingredients:

3 bacon slices

3 oz cream cheese

1 jalapeño pepper, chopped

½ tsp dried parsley

¼ tsp garlic powder

¼ tsp onion powder

Salt and ground black pepper to taste

Directions:

1. Preheat skillet on medium high heat.
2. Put bacon in skillet and cook until crispy.
3. Remove bacon from pan and place on paper towel. Crumble bacon. Reserve bacon fat from skillet.
4. Combine cream cheese with jalapeño pepper, parsley, garlic powder, onion powder, salt and black pepper.
5. Add bacon and bacon fat to jalapeño mixture. Stir gently.
6. Make balls and serve.

Nutrition per Serving: Calories - 198, Carbs – 1.98g, Fat – 19g, Protein – 4.9g

Breakfast Chia Seeds Porridge

Prep time: 10 minutes | Cook time: 12 minutes | Servings: 5

Ingredients:

8 oz coconut milk

8 oz almond milk

1 tbsp butter

4 tbsp chia seeds

1 oz macadamia nuts, crushed

2 oz pumpkin seeds

2 tbsp stevia

Directions:

1. In sauce pan, whisk together coconut milk and almond milk.
2. Preheat mixture on medium heat and add butter, stir until butter dissolved. Bring to boil.
3. Add chia seeds and stir. Bring to boil again.
4. In a medium bowl, mix together macadamia nuts and pumpkin seeds.
5. Decrease temperature to low heat. Add nut mixture and cook for 3 minutes. Stir it constantly.
6. When porridge is cooked, let it cool for 3 minutes.
7. Stir in stevia and transfer to serving bowl. Serve warm.

Nutrition per Serving: Calories - 351, Carbs – 7.9g, Fat - 35g, Protein - 5.7g

Cereal Nibs

Prep time: 15 minutes | Cook time: 50 minutes | Servings: 4

Ingredients:

1 cup water

½ cup chia seeds

1 tbsp psyllium powder

1 tbsp vanilla extract

2 tbsp coconut oil

4 tbsp hemp hearts

1 tbsp swerve

2 tbsp cocoa nibs

Directions:

1. Combine water with chia seeds. Mix well and set aside for 5 minutes.
2. Stir in psyllium powder, vanilla extract, oil, hemp hearts, and swerve. Mix well.
3. Add cocoa nibs and stir until get dough.
4. Divide dough into 2 pieces. Make two cylinders from dough.
5. Put cylinders on baking sheet, flatten and cover with parchment paper.
6. Preheat oven to 285 F.
7. Place baking sheet in oven and cook for 20 minutes.
8. Remove parchment paper and cook for 25 minutes more.
9. Let cylinders cool down and cut into small pieces. Serve.

Nutrition per Serving: Calories - 250, Carbs – 1.99g, Fat – 13g, Protein – 8.8g

Breakfast Green Smoothie

Prep time: 6 minutes | Cook time: 0 minutes | Servings: 1

Ingredients:

½ avocado, peeled and chopped

1½ cups almond milk

1 tbsp coconut oil

1 oz spinach, chopped

1 scoop vanilla protein powder

10 drops liquid stevia

Directions:

1. Place avocado, almond milk, coconut oil, and spinach in blender or food processor. Blend well.
2. Add vanilla and liquid stevia and blend until smooth.
3. Serve.

Nutrition per Serving: Calories – 498, Carbs – 3.9g, Fat – 38g, Protein – 29.7g

Blackberry Keto Muffins

Prep time: 15 minutes | Cook time: 22 minutes | Servings: 4

Ingredients:

1 large egg, beaten

¼ tsp salt

1 tbsp lemon juice

½ tsp baking soda

½ cup almond milk

½ cup blackberry

1 tsp stevia

1 cup coconut flour

1 tbsp butter

Directions:

1. In medium bowl, whisk egg with salt.
2. Add baking soda and lemon juice. Mix well.
3. Pour in almond milk and stir gently.
4. Place blackberries in blender or food processor and blend until texture is smooth.
5. Add stevia and blend it for another 10 seconds.
6. Combine blackberry mixture with egg mixture
7. Add coconut flour and knead the homogenous dough.
8. Grease muffins forms with butter.
9. Fill 1/3 of each muffins form with this dough.
10. Preheat oven to 365 F.
11. Place forms in oven and bake dish for 20 minutes.
12. Remove from oven and let muffins cool for 5 minutes.
13. Separate muffins from forms and serve.

Nutrition per Serving: Calories - 179, Carbs - 7.5g, Fat - 16g, Protein – 3.9g

Simple French Toast

Prep time: 10 minutes | Cook time: 50 minutes | Servings: 8

Ingredients:

12 egg whites

8 oz whey protein

4 oz cream cheese

For the French toast:

2 medium eggs, beaten

½ cup coconut milk

1 tsp ground cinnamon

1 tsp vanilla extract

4 oz butter

½ cup almond milk

½ cup swerve

Directions:

1. Using mixer, whisk 12 egg whites for 2-3 minutes.
2. Add protein and stir.
3. Add cream cheese and stir.
4. Preheat oven to 325 F.
5. Grease 2 bread pans. Pour egg mixture into pans.
6. Place them in oven and cook for 45 minutes.
7. Slice bread into 18 pieces.
8. In a bowl, whisk together 2 eggs, coconut milk, cinnamon, and vanilla extract.
9. Toss bread slices in this mixture.
10. Preheat pan with oil on medium heat. Put bread slices and cook on both sides until they are golden.
11. Add butter to pan and melt it. Add almond milk and heat up on high heat.
12. Add swerve and stir. Take off heat.
13. Set aside and let it cool. Pour this mixture over French toast. Serve.

Nutrition per Serving: Calories - 198, Carbs – 0.99g, Fat – 13g, Protein – 6.9g

Liver Mousse

Prep time: 15 minutes | Cook time: 25 minutes | Servings: 4

Ingredients:

10 oz chicken liver, washed

2 cups water

1 white onion, peeled and chopped

1 tsp salt

½ tsp ground black pepper

1 tbsp cream

1 tbsp butter

Directions:

1. Put chicken liver in saucepan and add water.
2. Bring water to boil, close lid, and cook for 10 minutes on medium heat.
3. Place onion in blender or food processor and blend until the texture is smooth.
4. Season onion with salt and pepper. Mix well.
5. Transfer onion mixture to a bowl.
6. Place cooked liver in blender and blend it too until smooth.
7. Mix together liver and onion mixture. Stir carefully.
8. Add cream and stir.
9. Grease baking form with butter and place liver mixture in it.
10. Set oven to 350 F and heat it up.
11. Transfer baking form to oven and bake liver mousse for 10 minutes.
12. When liver mousse is cooked, stir it carefully.
13. Let dish cool for 5 minutes and serve.

Nutrition per Serving: Calories - 160, Carbs - 4g, Fat - 8g, Protein - 18g

Waffles

Prep time: 15 minutes | Cook time: 25 minutes | Servings: 5

Ingredients:

5 medium eggs, separated

1 tsp baking powder

4 tbsp coconut flour

3 tbsp almond milk

4 oz butter, melted

3 tbsp stevia

2 tsp vanilla extract

Directions:

1. Using mixer, whisk egg whites.
2. In a medium bowl, combine egg yolks, baking powder, flour, milk, butter, stevia and vanilla extract. Mix well.
3. Add whisked egg whites and stir well.
4. Pour mixture into waffle maker and bake until it is golden.
5. You may have to do it in two-three batches.
6. Serve hot.

Nutrition per Serving: Calories - 238, Carbs – 3.97g, Fat – 22g, Protein – 6.9g

White Mushroom Frittata

Prep time: 20 minutes | Cook time: 25 minutes | Servings: 4

Ingredients:

5 medium eggs, beaten

6 oz white mushrooms, washed and sliced

1 tsp ghee

½ tsp salt

1 tsp paprika

1/3 tsp ground black pepper

5.5 oz asparagus, chopped

3 medium celery stalk, chopped

1 tsp chives, chopped

2 tbsp olive oil

½ cup white onion, chopped

Directions:

1. In a bowl, whisk eggs using mixer.
2. Add ghee, salt, paprika, and black pepper and mix well. Set aside.
3. In another bowl, combine asparagus, celery stalk and chives.
4. Preheat pan with 1 tablespoon of olive oil on medium heat.
5. Put mushrooms in pan and sauté for 2 minutes, stirring constantly.
6. Add vegetables mixture and sauté for another 3 minutes.
7. Add chopped onion and cook for 1 minute more, stirring constantly.
8. Pour in 1 tablespoon of olive oil and stir.
9. Pour egg mixture over vegetables and place pan in preheated on 365 F oven.
10. Cook frittata for 14 minutes. Serve warm.

Nutrition per Serving: Calories - 270, Carbs - 8g, Fat - 19g, Protein - 13g

Nutty Breakfast Smoothie

Prep time: 10 minutes | Cook time: 0 minutes | Servings: 1

Ingredients:

2 brazil nuts

2 cups spinach leaves

10 almonds

1 cup coconut milk

1 tbsp psyllium seeds

1 tsp greens powder

1 tbsp potato starch

1 tsp whey protein

Directions:

1. Place Brazil nuts, spinach, almonds, and coconut milk in a blender or food processor and blend well.
2. Add psyllium seeds, greens powder, potato starch, and protein, blend.
3. Pour mixture in glass. Serve.

Nutrition per Serving: Calories - 338, Carbs – 6.85g, Fat – 29g, Protein – 13g

Breakfast Coffee Shake

Prep time: 5 minutes | Cook time: 0 minutes | Servings: 1

Ingredients:

1 cup brewed coffee

1 scoop vanilla protein powder (about 30 grams)

1 tbsp coconut oil

¼ cup heavy cream

Directions:

1. Pour brewed coffee in blender or food processor.
2. Add protein powder, coconut oil and heavy cream.
3. Blend mass for 20 seconds on high.
4. Serve.

Nutrition per Serving: Calories – 420, Carbs – 1.1g, Fat – 37.7g, Protein – 24.8g

Low Carb Chicken Quesadilla

Prep time: 15 minutes | Cook time: 7 minutes | Servings: 1 quesadilla

Ingredients:

2½ oz chicken breast, grilled

1 low carb wrap

3 oz pepper jack

1 tsp jalapeño, chopped

½ avocado, sliced thin

Spices for chicken:

¼ tsp garlic powder

¼ tsp dried basil

¼ tsp salt

¼ tsp crushed red pepper

Directions:

1. Chop and grill chicken with spices mix.
2. Preheat pan on medium heat and place low carb wrap on pan.
3. Heat wrap for 2 minutes, then flip and put pepper jack on wrap.
4. Add chopped jalapeño, avocado and chicken to one half of wrap.
5. Fold wrap over: use spatula to lift up one side of wrap and flip over other side.
6. Take pan off heat and serve with the lettuce, salsa, sour cream, and guacamole.

Nutrition per Serving: Calories - 649, Carbs – 6.9g, Fat – 42.8g, Protein – 51.5g

Chicken Quiche

Prep time: 15 minutes | Cook time: 50 minutes | Servings: 6

Ingredients:

16 oz almond flour

7 medium eggs

Salt and ground black pepper to taste

2 tbsp coconut oil

1 lb ground chicken

2 small zucchini, grated

1 tsp dried oregano

1 tsp fennel seeds

½ cup heavy cream

Directions:

1. Place almond flour, 1 egg, salt and coconut oil in blender or food processor and blend.
2. Grease pie pan and pour dough in it. Press well on bottom.
3. Preheat pan on medium heat and toss ground chicken, cook for 2 minutes, set aside.
4. In medium bowl, whisk together 6 eggs, zucchini, oregano, salt, pepper, fennel seeds and heavy cream.
5. Add chicken to egg mixture and stir well.
6. Preheat oven to 350 F.
7. Pour egg mixture into pie pan and place in oven. Cook for 40 minutes.
8. Let it cool and slice. Serve.

Nutrition per Serving: Calories - 295, Carbs – 3.95g, Fat – 24g, Protein – 19g

Chicken Pancakes

Prep time: 15 minutes | Cook time: 10 minutes | Servings: 6

Ingredients:

3 medium eggs, beaten

½ tsp salt

1 tsp rosemary

1 tsp basil

½ cup almond milk

3 tbsp coconut flour

2 oz almond flour

6 oz ground chicken

2 tbsp butter

Directions:

1. Season eggs with salt, rosemary, basil, and almond milk.
2. Whisk mixture with hand mixer to get homogenous texture.
3. Add coconut and almond flour. Mix until you get smooth batter.
4. Add chicken and stir carefully.
5. Heat up pan with butter and melt it.
6. ladle about 1/4 cup of batter onto pan, to make pancake. Make 1 or 2 more pancakes, taking care to keep them evenly spaced apart.
7. Bake pancakes for 1 minute on each side until golden brown.
8. Serve hot.

Nutrition per Serving: Calories - 199, Carbs - 3.8g, Fat - 16g, Protein - 13g

Cheddar Chicken and Broccoli Casserole

Prep time: 35 minutes | Cook time: 28 minutes | Servings: 4

Ingredients:

2 cups broccoli, divided into florets and steamed (or frozen)

20 oz chicken breast, cooked and shredded

½ cup sour cream

2 tbsp olive oil

½ cup heavy cream

Salt and ground black pepper to taste

1 tsp oregano

½ tsp paprika

1 cup cheddar cheese, shredded

1 oz pork rinds, crushed

Directions:

1. Set oven to 450 F and heat it up.
2. In medium bowl, mix together broccoli, chicken, sour cream and olive oil.
3. Grease baking form, add chicken mixture to it and press to bottom.
4. Spread heavy cream over chicken layer.
5. Season with salt, black pepper, oregano and paprika.
6. Top with shredded cheese.
7. Sprinkle dish with crushed pork rinds.
8. Place in oven and cook for 20-25 minutes until dish edges browned.
9. Serve with marinara sauce.

Nutrition per Serving: Calories – 550, Carbs – 3.9g, Fat – 41.8g, Protein – 43.5g

Italian Chicken

Prep time: 15 minutes | Cook time: 25 minutes | Servings: 6

Ingredients:

Salt and ground black pepper to taste

¼ cup olive oil

4 chicken breasts, skinless and boneless

4 cloves garlic

½ cup green olives, pitted and chopped

4 anchovy fillets, chopped

1 medium onion

1 tbsp capers, chopped

½ tsp red chili flakes

1 lb tomatoes, cored and chopped

Directions:

1. In bowl, mix together salt, pepper and 1/8 cup of olive oil.
2. Rub chicken breasts with this mixture.
3. Heat up pan over high heat.
4. Put chicken in pan and cook for 2 minutes on each side.
5. Preheat oven to 450 F.
6. Put pan with chicken in oven and cook for 8 minutes.
7. Transfer cooked chicken breasts to serving bowl.
8. Heat up pan with rest of oil over medium heat.
9. Peel and chop garlic and onion.
10. Add garlic, olives, anchovies, onion, capers, and chili flakes, cook for 1 minute stirring occasionally
11. Season with pepper and salt, stir.
12. Add tomatoes, stir and cook for another 2 minutes.
13. Pour sauce over chicken breasts and serve.

Nutrition per Serving: Calories - 394, Carbs – 2.1g, Fat – 19.8g, Protein – 6.95g

Tasty Chicken with Mushrooms

Prep time: 20 minutes | Cook time: 47 minutes | Servings: 1

Ingredients:

2 tbsp butter

8 oz white mushrooms, chopped

¼ cup water

1 tsp fresh lemon juice

¼ cup heavy cream

Salt and ground black pepper to taste

6 oz chicken breast, cooked

1 handful of spinach

Directions:

1. Preheat pan on medium heat and melt butter.
2. Add mushrooms and sauté until crisped up.
3. Pour in water and lemon juice, stir.
4. Add heavy cream, stir and cook until sauce thickened.
5. Sprinkle with salt and black pepper and add cooked chicken breasts.
6. Serve with spinach.

Nutrition per Serving: Calories - 637, Carbs – 4.9g, Fat – 49.8g, Protein – 45.5g

Chicken-Stuffed Avocados

Prep time: 15 minutes | Cook time: 0 minutes | Servings: 2

Ingredients:

2 avocados

12 oz chicken, cooked and shredded

2 tbsp lemon juice

2 tbsp cream cheese

¼ cup mayonnaise

½ tsp garlic powder

½ tsp onion powder

1 tsp dried thyme

Salt and ground black pepper to taste

1 tsp paprika

¼ tsp cayenne pepper

Directions:

1. Cut avocados in half and remove the pits.
2. Scoop out avocado insides, and put flesh in a bowl.
3. Save empty avocado halves.
4. Combine avocado flesh with shredded chicken.
5. Stir in lemon juice, cream cheese, mayonnaise, garlic powder, onion powder, thyme, salt, pepper, paprika, and cayenne pepper. Mix well.
6. Divide chicken mixture among avocado halves and serve.

Nutrition per Serving: Calories - 225, Carbs – 4.9g, Fat – 39g, Protein – 23g

Pan-seared Duck Breast

Prep time: 15 minutes | Cook time: 25 minutes | Servings: 1

Ingredients:

2 tbsp butter

1 tbsp swerve

¼ tsp fresh sage

½ tsp orange extract

1 tbsp heavy cream

1 medium duck breast, skin scored

1 cup baby spinach

Salt and ground black pepper to taste

Directions:

1. Preheat saucepan on medium heat and add butter, melt it.
2. Pour in swerve, stir and cook until butter browns.
3. Add sage and orange extract to pan, stir, and sauté for 2 minutes.
4. Add cream and mix well.
5. Preheat another pan on medium high heat.
6. Put duck in pan, skin side down, cook for 4 minutes on one side. Then flip and cook for 3 minutes on other side.
7. Pour some orange mixture over breast and stir. Cook for 2 minutes more.
8. Add spinach, salt and pepper to saucepan, stir and cook for 1 minute.
9. When duck is cooked, slice breast.
10. Pour orange sauce over sliced duck breast and serve.

Nutrition per Serving: Calories - 558, Carbs – 0.8g, Fat – 54g, Protein – 37g

Chicken Skillet

Prep time: 20 minutes | Cook time: 35 minutes | Servings: 4

Ingredients:

12 oz chicken fillet, cut into strips

1 tsp salt

½ tsp ground black pepper

1 tsp cilantro

1 tsp oregano

1 tsp basil

¼ tsp chili pepper

¼ cup cream cheese

6 oz white mushrooms, sliced

2 tbsp coconut oil

½ cup spinach

1 white onion

Directions:

1. In medium bowl, combine chicken strips with salt, black pepper, cilantro, oregano, basil, and chili pepper.
2. In another bowl, mix together cream cheese and mushrooms.
3. Heat up pan with coconut oil over medium heat.
4. Put chicken on pan and cook for 10 minutes
5. Chop spinach and mix with mushroom and cheese mixture.
6. Add this mixture to pan and close lid. Cook for 15 minutes more.
7. Meanwhile, peel and chop onion.
8. Add onion to pan and cook for another 5 minutes.
9. Stir cooked dish gently and serve.

Nutrition per Serving: Calories - 338, Carbs - 5g, Fat - 25g, Protein - 28g

Chicken Zucchini Noodles Soup

Prep time: 25 minutes | Cook time: 57 minutes | Servings: 3

Ingredients:

2 tbsp olive oil

½ medium white onion, chopped

1 stalk celery, chopped

1 medium carrot, chopped

1 tbsp dried oregano

Salt and ground black pepper to taste

4 cups chicken broth

8 oz chicken thighs, boneless and skinless

1 large zucchini

¼ cup sour cream

Directions:

1. Preheat pot with oil on medium heat, add onion and sauté for 2-3 minutes or until translucent.
2. Add chopped celery, carrots, oregano, black pepper and salt. Continue sauté until slightly softened.
3. Pour in chicken broth and bring mixture to boil.
4. Add chicken thighs, lower heat and simmer for 30 minutes.
5. Take out chicken from pot and shred meat.
6. Add shredded chicken back to pot and cook for 15 minutes more.
7. Meanwhile, using spiralizer, make zucchini noodles.
8. Add to soup and cook for another 2-3 minutes.
9. Serve hot with sour cream.

Nutrition per Serving: Calories – 368, Carbs – 7.85g, Fat – 25.5g, Protein – 22.9g

Roasted Pork Belly

Prep time: 15 minutes | Cook time: 1 hour 40 minutes | Servings: 8

Ingredients:

18 oz apples, cored, and cut into wedges

2 tbsp stevia

4 cups water

1 tbsp lemon juice

2 lbs pork belly, scored

Salt and ground black pepper to taste

A drizzle of olive oil

Directions:

1. Place apples, stevia, water and lemon juice in blender or food processor and blend them well.
2. Steam pork for 1 hour in steamer tray.
3. Rub pork with salt, pepper and olive oil.
4. Put pork belly on baking sheet and drizzle apple sauce on top.
5. Preheat oven to 425 F.
6. Place baking sheet in oven and cook for 30 minutes.
7. Slice pork and serve with apple sauce.

Nutrition per Serving: Calories - 461, Carbs – 11g, Fat – 35g, Protein – 26g

Soft and Juicy Pork Cutlets

Prep time: 15 minutes | Cook time: 15 minutes | Servings: 2

Ingredients:

2 tbsp butter

10 oz ground pork

1 tsp salt

1 tsp rosemary

1 tbsp oregano

1 tsp paprika

½ tsp turmeric

2 eggs

2 tsp coconut oil

1 tbsp almond flour

Directions:

1. In bowl, mix together butter and pork.
2. Season with salt, rosemary, oregano, paprika, and turmeric, stir well with hands.
3. Shape cutlets and set aside.
4. In another bowl, whisk eggs until get homogenous texture.
5. Heat up pan with coconut oil over medium heat.
6. Dip pork cutlets in egg mixture and sprinkle with almond flour.
7. Place cutlets on pan and cook for 7 minutes on both sides.
8. Transfer cutlets to paper towel and drain grease.
9. Serve warm.

Nutrition per Serving: Calories - 390, Carbs - 1.2g, Fat - 21g, Protein - 41g

Green Beans and Mustard Lemon Pork

Prep time: 20 minutes | Cook time: 12 minutes | Servings: 1

Ingredients:

2 4-oz pork loin

1 tsp thyme

1 tsp paprika

1 tsp black pepper

1 tbsp pink Himalayan sea salt

1 tbsp olive oil

1 cup green beans

Mustard Sauce

2 tbsp heavy cream

½ tsp apple cider vinegar

½ cup chicken broth

½ tbsp mustard

Juice from ¼ lemon

Directions:

1. Wash pork loin and pat dry with kitchen paper towel.
2. In mixing bowl, mix together thyme, paprika, black pepper, and salt.
3. Rub pork loin with spice mixture.
4. Heat up pan over high heat and add olive oil. Put pork in pan and cook for 2 minutes on both sides.
5. Remove meat from pan.
6. Add heavy cream, apple cider vinegar and broth in pan and deglaze it by scraping the bottom to remove all of the brown bits.
7. Bring broth mixture to simmer.
8. Add mustard and lemon juice, stir.
9. Add pork loin back to pan and stir to coat meat with sauce.
10. Close lid and cook for 10 minutes (you can left lid slightly open).
11. Preheat oven to 350 F. Roast green beans in oven for 10 minutes.
12. Serve pork loin sauce with green beans.

Nutrition per Serving: Calories – 588, Carbs – 3.9g, Fat – 44g, Protein – 50g

Fried Cheese in Bacon Strips

Prep time: 15 minutes | Cook time: 15 minutes | Servings: 4

Ingredients:

2 eggs, beaten

½ tsp ground black pepper

1 tsp oregano

10 oz Cheddar cheese, cubed

7 oz bacon strips

1 tbsp almond flour

5 tbsp butter

1 tsp salt

Directions:

1. Whisk eggs until you get smooth and homogenous mass.
2. Season with black pepper and oregano. Mix well.
3. In bowl, combine salt and bacon.
4. Wrap Cheddar cheese cubes in bacon strips.
5. Dip wrapped cheese in egg mixture and dust with almond flour.
6. Prepare 5 muffin forms and add butter in each form.
7. Put bacon wraps in forms.
8. Place muffin forms in oven at 370 F, and bake for 10 minutes.
9. Let dish cool for 5 minutes and serve.

Nutrition per Serving: Calories - 537, Carbs – 2.98g, Fat - 48.8g, Protein – 22.9g

Beef Meatball Casserole

Prep time: 15 minutes | Cook time: 55 minutes | Servings: 8

Ingredients:

1 lb ground beef

1 lb beef sausage, chopped

Salt and ground black pepper to taste

⅓ cup almond flour

2 eggs, beaten

½ tsp garlic powder

¼ tsp onion powder

¼ cup Parmesan cheese, grated

¼ tsp dried oregano

¼ tsp red pepper flakes

1 tbsp dried parsley

2 cups keto marinara sauce

1 cup ricotta cheese

1½ cups mozzarella cheese, shredded

Directions:

1. In medium bowl, combine ground beef, sausage, salt and pepper.
2. Add almond flour, eggs, garlic powder and onion powder, stir well.
3. Sprinkle with Parmesan cheese, oregano, pepper flakes, and parsley, mix well.
4. Make meatballs with your hands and put them on baking sheet.
5. Preheat oven to 375 F. Place baking sheet in it and cook for 15 minutes.
6. Transfer meatballs to baking dish, sprinkle with ricotta cheese and pour marinara sauce over dish.
7. Season with mozzarella and place dish in oven at 375 F. Cook for 30 minutes more.
8. Let cooked meatballs cool and serve.

Nutrition per Serving: Calories – 449, Carbs – 3.98g, Fat – 34g, Protein – 31g

Roasted Meat Mixture

Prep time: 20 minutes | Cook time: 50 minutes | Servings: 8

Ingredients:

1 tbsp oregano

1 tsp cayenne pepper

1 tsp basil

1 tsp salt

7 oz beef brisket, cut into strips

8 oz lamb, cut into strips

3 oz pork, cut into strips

5 oz chicken, cut into strips

4 tbsp butter

2 cups water

6 oz asparagus, chopped

1 white onion, peeled and diced

Directions:

1. In medium bowl, combine oregano, cayenne pepper, basil and salt.
2. Rub meat strips with spice mixture and set aside.
3. Heat up skillet over medium heat, add and melt butter.
4. Put meat strips on skillet and cook on high heat for 4-5 minutes, stirring constantly.
5. Transfer meat to pan and add water.
6. Add onion and asparagus, stir carefully.
7. Simmer meat mixture on medium heat for 40 minutes.
8. Serve warm.

Nutrition per Serving: Calories - 229, Carbs – 2.98g, Fat – 12.4g, Protein - 28.2g

Steak and Eggs

Prep time: 12 minutes | Cook time: 6 minutes | Servings: 1

Ingredients:

1 tbsp olive oil

4 oz sirloin

1 tbsp butter

Salt and ground black pepper to taste

3 large eggs, beaten

½ avocado, peeled and sliced

Directions:

1. Preheat pan with oil on medium heat.
2. Add sirloin and cook until desired doneness.
3. Transfer to plate, sprinkle with salt and pepper and slice meat into bite-sized.
4. Melt butter in pan and add eggs. Cook for 3-5 minutes or until desired doneness.
5. Serve sliced meat with eggs and avocado.

Nutrition per Serving: Calories – 690, Carbs – 4.8g, Fat – 53g, Protein – 42.9g

Spicy Beef Steak

Prep time: 20 minutes | Cook time: 35 minutes | Servings: 4

Ingredients:

16 oz beef steak

1 tbsp rosemary

1 tsp basil

1 tsp ground black pepper

Salt to taste

1 tsp cilantro

1 tsp turmeric

1 tsp oregano

1 tsp mustard

1 tsp apple cider vinegar

1 tbsp lemon juice

1 tbsp coconut oil

1 tbsp almond milk

2 tbsp butter

Directions:

1. Beat beef steaks gently.
2. In medium bowl, mix together rosemary, basil, black pepper, salt, cilantro, turmeric, and oregano.
3. Rub all sides of beef steaks with spice mixture.
4. Then rub with mustard and drizzle with apple cider vinegar and lemon juice.
5. Set aside for 5 minutes.
6. In another bowl, mix together coconut oil, almond milk, and butter.
7. Heat up pan over medium heat and add coconut oil mixture
8. Put meat in pan and cook for 15 minutes on both sides.
9. Serve hot.

Nutrition per Serving: Calories - 401, Carbs – 2.8g, Fat - 23g, Protein - 44g

Sriracha Lime Flank Steak

Prep time: 10 minutes | Cook time: 17 minutes | Servings: 1

Ingredients:

1 tbsp olive oil

7 oz asparagus, ends trimmed off

8 oz flank steak

Salt and ground black pepper to taste

Sriracha Lime Sauce:

1 tbsp sriracha

Juice from ½ lime

Salt and ground black pepper to taste

1 tbsp olive oil

½ tsp vinegar

Directions:

1. Preheat pan with olive oil on medium heat.
2. Add asparagus and cook for 10 minutes, stirring occasionally. Transfer to bowl, cover and set aside.
3. Rub flank steak with black pepper and salt.
4. Put in pan and brown for 6-7 minutes per side.
5. Meanwhile, in bowl combine sriracha, lime juice, salt, black pepper, olive oil and vinegar. Stir well until sauce is thickened.
6. When steak is done, slice it and serve with asparagus and sauce.

Nutrition per Serving: Calories – 554, Carbs – 7.9g, Fat – 35g, Protein – 53.2g

Beef Stew

Prep time: 25 minutes | Cook time: 45 minutes | Servings: 6

Ingredients:

1 tsp salt

½ tsp ground black pepper

1 tbsp mustard

1 tsp paprika

1 tsp rosemary

1 lb beef brisket, cut into 1½ inch cubes

10 oz asparagus

7 oz avocado, pitted and peeled

2 cups beef broth

¼ cup cream cheese

1/3 oz flax meal

1 oz walnuts, crushed

Directions:

1. In medium bowl, mix together salt, black pepper, mustard, paprika, and rosemary.
2. Put meat cubes in bowl and rub with spice mixture. Set aside
3. Cut asparagus into 4 parts and chop avocado.
4. Pour beef broth into saucepan and heat up over medium-high heat.
5. Bring beef broth to boil and toss beef brisket in it. Simmer for 15 minutes on medium heat.
6. Add asparagus and cook for another 15 minutes.
7. Meanwhile, combine cream cheese with avocado. Add flax meal and stir carefully.
8. Add mixture to meat stew and stir gently to get homogenous mass.
9. Cover with lid and cook for 10 minutes more.
10. Top with crushed walnuts and serve.

Nutrition per Serving: Calories - 309, Carbs - 7.4g, Fat – 18.9g, Protein - 28g

Quick Asian Crack Slaw

Prep time: 15 minutes | Cook time: 17 minutes | Servings: 2

Ingredients:

1 tbsp sesame seed oil

1 garlic clove, minced

½ lb ground beef

5 oz coleslaw salad mix

1 tbsp soy sauce

1 tbsp olive oil

1 tsp sesame seeds

Salt and ground black pepper to taste

1 stalk green onion, chopped

Directions:

1. Preheat large wok with sesame seed oil, add minced garlic and cook for 1-2 minutes, until fragrant.
2. Add beef and stir well. Brown for 5-10 minutes, stirring occasionally.
3. Toss coleslaw salad mix in wok and stir.
4. Pour soy sauce and olive oil in wok, stir and cook for 5 minutes more.
5. Sprinkle with black pepper, sesame seeds and black pepper.
6. Top with green onion and serve.

Nutrition per Serving: Calories – 368, Carbs – 3.9g, Fat – 26.5g, Protein – 23.9g

Steak Bowl

Prep time: 20 minutes | Cook time: 12 minutes | Servings: 3

Ingredients:

½ cup fresh cilantro

4 oz pepper jack cheese

16 oz skirt steak

Salt and ground black pepper to taste

1 cup sour cream

A splash of chipotle adobo sauce

For the guacamole:

2 avocados, pitted and peeled

Salt and ground black pepper to taste

6 cherry tomatoes, cored and chopped

1 clove garlic, peeled and minced

¼ cup onion, chopped

Juice from 1 lime

1 tbsp olive oil

1 tbsp fresh cilantro

Directions:

1. Chop cilantro and shred pepper jack cheese.
2. In medium bowl, mash avocado with fork and add salt, black pepper, tomatoes, garlic, and onion. Mix well.
3. Pour in lime juice and olive oil.
4. Chop cilantro and add to lime mixture, mix well.
5. Preheat pan on high heat. Add steak, sprinkle with salt and pepper and brown for 8 minutes on both sides. Transfer to serving plate and cut into thin strips.
6. Top with cheese, sour cream and guacamole. Drizzle with chipotle adobo sauce.
7. Serve.

Nutrition per Serving: Calories - 597, Carbs – 4.95g, Fat – 49g, Protein – 29g

Meatball Pilaf

Prep time: 15 minutes | Cook time: 35 minutes | Servings: 4

Ingredients:

12 oz cauliflower, divided into florets

1 cup cooked rice

2 tbsp coconut oil

Salt and ground black pepper to taste

1 lb ground lamb

1 egg, beaten

1 tsp garlic powder

1 tsp paprika

1 tsp fennel seed

1 onion,

2 cloves garlic

1 tbsp lemon zest

1 bunch fresh mint, chopped

4 oz goat cheese, crumbled

Directions:

1. Place cauliflower florets in blender or food processor and blend well.
2. In bowl, combine rice with cauliflower.
3. Preheat pan with 1 tbsp of coconut oil on medium heat.
4. Put cauliflower rice on pan and cook for 8 minutes; sprinkle with pepper and salt, stir and set aside.
5. In another bowl, combine lamb, egg, garlic powder, paprika, black pepper, salt, and fennel seed.
6. Make 12 meatballs and set aside.
7. Preheat pan with 1 tbsp of coconut oil on medium heat.
8. Peel and chop onion. Peel and mince garlic.
9. Add onion and sauté for 6 minutes until golden.
10. Add garlic and sauté for 1 minute more.
11. Put meatballs in pan and brown them on all sides well.
12. Serve meatballs with cauliflower rice and top with lemon zest, fresh mint and goat cheese.

Nutrition per Serving: Calories - 469, Carbs – 3.9g, Fat – 44g, Protein – 25g

Crunchy Bacon Casserole

Prep time: 25 minutes | Cook time: 45 minutes | Servings: 3

Ingredients:

2 eggs, beaten

1/3 cup almond milk

1 tsp turmeric

1 tsp salt

1 cup ground pork

2 tbsp butter

¼ cup asparagus, chopped

¼ cup green beans

1 zucchini

½ cup Parmesan cheese, grated

Directions:

1. In mixer, mix together eggs, almond milk, turmeric and salt.
2. In medium bowl, combine ground pork and butter.
3. Put ground pork mixture in baking form.
4. Add asparagus and green beans.
5. Slice zucchini and place on top.
6. Pour almond mixture over zucchini.
7. Sprinkle with Parmesan cheese.
8. Cover the pan tightly with aluminum foil.
9. Transfer dish to oven at 365 F, and bake for 25 minutes.
10. Then remove aluminum foil and bake casserole for another 15 minutes.
11. Let it cool 5 minutes and serve.

Nutrition per Serving: Calories - 320, Carbs – 4.99g, Fat - 21g, Protein – 27.95g

Low Carb Bunless Butter Burger

Prep time: 10 minutes | Cook time: 17 minutes | Servings: 1

Ingredients:

½ cup ground beef

1 tsp paprika

Salt and ground black pepper to taste

1 tbsp butter

1 tbsp olive oil

1 large leaf of lettuce

1 slice cheese

1 tsp mayonnaise

Directions:

1. In small bowl, combine beef with paprika, black pepper and salt. Mix up well.
2. Shape meat mixture into 2 flat patties.
3. Put butter in center of each patty.
4. Put second patty on top of first patty and press until both patties merge.
5. Preheat pan with oil on high heat. Add patty for 4 minutes per side.
6. Transfer patty to lettuce leaf and top with cheese.
7. Spread mayonnaise and fold lettuce leaf.
8. Serve.

Nutrition per Serving: Calories – 635, Carbs – 1.1g, Fat – 60g, Protein – 23.8g

Avocado Tuna Salad

Prep time: 18 minutes | Cook time: 0 minutes | Servings: 1

Ingredients:

½ avocado, peeled and chopped

4 oz canned tuna

½ stalk celery, diced

½ tsp fresh lemon juice

1 tsp mustard

2 tbsp mayonnaise

Salt and ground black pepper to taste

1 big hard-boiled egg, peeled and chopped

Directions:

1. In mixing bowl, mix together avocado, tuna and celery.
2. Add lemon juice, mustard, and mayonnaise, stir.
3. Sprinkle with salt and black pepper.
4. Add chopped egg and stir well.
5. Serve.

Nutrition per Serving: Calories – 511, Carbs – 5.1g, Fat – 33.7g, Protein – 30g

Easy Stuffed Avocado

Prep time: 15 minutes | Cook time: 0 minutes | Servings: 2

Ingredients:

1 avocado, cut in half

½ cup canned sardines, drained

1 tbsp lemon juice

1 tbsp mayonnaise

¼ tsp turmeric

1 green onion, peeled and chopped

Salt and ground black pepper to taste

Directions:

1. Scoop out avocado insides and save empty avocado halves.
2. In bowl, combine avocado flesh with sardines and mash with fork.
3. Add lemon juice, mayonnaise, turmeric, onion, pepper and salt, mix well.
4. Divide mixture among avocado halves and serve.

Nutrition per Serving: Calories - 229, Carbs – 4.99g, Fat – 35g, Protein – 26.8g

Salmon Rolls

Prep time: 15 minutes | Cook time: 10 minutes | Servings: 3

Ingredients:

1 tbsp butter

½ cup cream cheese

1 tbsp oregano

1 tsp cilantro

1 tsp salt

1 tbsp dill

½ tsp garlic, minced

1 oz walnuts, crushed

1 tsp nutmeg

10 oz smoked salmon, sliced

Directions:

1. In medium bowl, using mixer, combine butter and cream cheese until smooth and fluffy.
2. Add oregano, cilantro, salt, dill, garlic and walnuts, stir carefully.
3. Add nutmeg and stir until you get homogenous mass.
4. Put this cream mixture on each salmon slice and roll them.
5. Place salmon rolls in fridge and wait for 10 minutes.
6. Take out rolls from fridge and serve.

Nutrition per Serving: Calories - 349, Carbs – 3.98g, Fat – 26.9g, Protein – 23.1g

Salmon and Cauli-rice with Avocado Lime Sauce

Prep time: 15 minutes | Cook time: 27 minutes | Servings: 1

Ingredients:

1½ oz cauliflower

Olive oil

½ avocado, peeled and chopped

1 tbsp red onion, peeled and diced

Juice of ½ lime

1 (6 oz) salmon fillet

Salt and ground black pepper to taste

Directions:

1. Place cauliflower in blender or food processor. Pulse about 14-18 times (short, quick pulses), until you get very small pieces.
2. Preheat pan with some olive oil on medium heat. Add cauli-rice and cook for 8 minutes, stirring occasionally.
3. Place avocado, onion and lime juice in blender or food processor and blend until smooth.
4. Preheat another pan with some oil on medium heat. Add fish fillet skin-side down, sprinkle with salt and pepper and cook for 4-5 minutes.
5. Flip fillet and cook for 4 minutes more.
6. Serve salmon fillet with cooked cauli-rice and avocado lime sauce.

Nutrition per Serving: Calories – 418, Carbs – 4.9g, Fat – 26.8g, Protein – 36.8g

Crab Rissoles

Prep time: 15 minutes | Cook time: 10 minutes | Servings: 5

Ingredients:

12 oz crab meat

2 eggs, beaten

1 tbsp flax meal

1 tsp onion powder

2 tbsp butter

1 tsp salt

1 tsp ground black pepper

1 tsp chives

1 tsp nutmeg

¼ cup almond milk

1 tbsp coconut flour

1 tbsp almond flour

1 tbsp coconut oil

Directions:

1. Cut crab meat into tiny pieces.
2. In bowl, combine eggs with crab meat, stir to get homogenous mass.
3. Add flax meal, onion powder, butter, salt, and black pepper, stir.
4. Add chives and nutmeg. Mix carefully.
5. Make medium rissoles and dip in almond milk.
6. In bowl, mix together coconut flour and almond flour.
7. Season rissoles with flour mixture.
8. Heat up skillet with coconut oil over medium heat.
9. Fry rissoles for 4 minutes on both sides.
10. Let them cool for 2-3 minutes and serve.

Nutrition per Serving: Calories - 229, Carbs – 5.98g, Fat - 18g, Protein – 12.95g

Baked Halibut with Vegetables

Prep time: 15 minutes | Cook time: 30 minutes | Servings: 2

Ingredients:

1 yellow bell pepper, seeded

1 red bell pepper, seeded

1 tbsp olive oil

Salt and ground black pepper to taste

1 tsp balsamic vinegar

2 halibut fillets

1 tsp cumin

2 cups baby spinach

Directions:

1. Chop bell peppers.
2. In mixing bowl, combine bell peppers, ½ tbsp of olive oil, black pepper, salt and vinegar.
3. Preheat oven to 400 F.
4. Put bell peppers mixture in baking dish and place in oven. Cook for 20 minutes.
5. Meanwhile, preheat pan with ½ tbsp oil on medium heat.
6. Put fish on pan, sprinkle with salt, pepper and cumin. Cook on both sides until browned.
7. Remove baked bell peppers from oven and add spinach, stir gently.
8. Serve fish on plate with vegetables.

Nutrition per Serving: Calories - 229, Carbs – 3.98g, Fat – 11.9g, Protein – 8.8g

Fried Calamari with Spicy Sauce

Prep time: 15 minutes | Cook time: 25 minutes | Servings: 2

Ingredients:

Salt and ground black pepper to taste

¼ tsp cayenne pepper

1 squid, cut into medium rings

1 egg, whisked

2 tbsp coconut flour

½ tbsp coconut oil

1 tsp sriracha sauce

4 tbsp mayonnaise

1 tbsp lemon juice

Directions:

1. In bowl, mix black pepper, salt, and cayenne pepper and rub squid rings with this mixture.
2. Whisk together egg, coconut flour, salt and black pepper.
3. Dip squid rings in egg mixture.
4. Preheat pan on medium heat and add coconut oil.
5. Put squid rings on pan and fry them on both sides until golden brown.
6. Transfer to paper towels and drain grease.
7. In medium bowl, combine sriracha sauce, mayonnaise and lemon juice.
8. Serve calamari rings with spicy sauce.

Nutrition per Serving: Calories – 351, Carbs – 2.9g, Fat – 31.8g, Protein – 12.8g

Spicy Grilled Shrimps

Prep time: 17 minutes | Cook time: 7 minutes | Servings: 2

Ingredients:

3 tbsp butter

1 tbsp garlic, minced

¼ tbsp turmeric

1 tsp cilantro

1 tsp basil

1 tsp rosemary

1 tsp oregano

15 oz shrimps, peeled

1 tsp salt

1 tbsp hot chili pepper

1 tbsp lemon juice

2 tbsp coconut oil

Directions:

1. In small bowl, combine together butter and garlic.
2. In medium bowl, mix together turmeric, cilantro, basil, rosemary, and oregano.
3. Season shrimp with salt.
4. Add shrimps to spice mixture and stir gently.
5. Add hot chili pepper and lemon juice and stir again.
6. Set aside for 10 minutes.
7. Heat up grill on medium heat.
8. Sprinkle shrimps with coconut oil and transfer to grill.
9. Cook for 3 minutes.
10. Sprinkle shrimps with ½ of butter mixture and cook for another 2 minutes.
11. Transfer cooked shrimps to serving bowl and pour remaining butter mixture over them.
12. Serve.

Nutrition per Serving: Calories - 359, Carbs - 5g, Fat – 22.9g, Protein: 33g

Shrimp and Mushroom Zucchini Pasta

Prep time: 20 minutes | Cook time: 45 minutes | Servings: 1

Ingredients:

1 tbsp olive oil

8 oz white mushrooms, sliced

1 tbsp butter

6 oz large shrimps, peeled

1 large zucchini

¼ cup marinara sauce

Salt and ground black pepper to taste

2 tbsp Parmesan cheese, shredded

Directions:

1. Preheat pan with oil on medium heat.
2. Add mushrooms and sauté until they have absorbed most of oil.
3. Toss butter in pan and continue cook until mushrooms have turned slightly golden.
4. Add shrimps and cook on both sides for 4 minutes more.
5. Meanwhile, using spiralizer, make zucchini noodles.
6. Add noodles to pan and cook for another 2 minutes.
7. Add marinara sauce and sprinkle with black pepper and salt. Stir gently.
8. Top with shredded Parmesan cheese and serve.

Nutrition per Serving: Calories – 496, Carbs – 7.4g, Fat – 31.8g, Protein – 43.7g

Trout with Pecan and Walnuts

Prep time: 20 minutes | Cook time: 20 minutes | Servings: 6

Ingredients:

1 oz pecan, crushed

1 oz walnuts, crushed

1 tsp oregano

1 tsp basil

½ tsp rosemary

1 tsp turmeric

3 lbs trout, cut into 6 filets

1 tsp sea salt

2 tbsp butter

1 tbsp orange juice

3 tbsp almond milk

3 cloves garlic, peeled and sliced

Directions:

1. In medium bowl, combine pecan, walnuts, oregano, basil, rosemary and turmeric. Stir well.
2. Season fish with salt.
3. Preheat pan on medium heat and melt butter.
4. Put fillets on pan and cook them on high heat from both sides until get crusty crunch.
5. Sprinkle fillets with orange juice and almond milk.
6. Place garlic cloves on fish fillets and cook fish for 4 minutes on medium heat.
7. Flip fillets and sprinkle with nut mixture, close lid and cook for another 5 minutes.
8. Serve warm.

Nutrition per Serving: Calories - 549, Carbs - 3g, Fat – 30.9g, Protein - 63g

Italian Clams Delight

Prep time: 15 minutes | Cook time: 15 minutes | Servings: 6

Ingredients:

½ cup butter

5 cloves garlic

16 oz white wine

36 clams, scrubbed

1 tsp red pepper flakes

2 tsp dried oregano

1 tsp fresh parsley, chopped

Directions:

1. Preheat pan on medium heat and melt butter.
2. Peel and mince garlic. Cook for 1 minute, stirring occasionally.
3. Pour in wine and stir.
4. Add pepper flakes, oregano and parsley, stir well.
5. Add clams and stir. Close lid and cook for 10 minutes.
6. When time is up, remove unopened clams and transfer clam mixture into serving bowl.
7. Serve.

Nutrition per Serving: Calories - 219, Carbs – 2.9g, Fat – 14.9g, Protein – 3.95g

Mackerel Bombs

Prep time: 15 minutes | Cook time: 10 minutes | Servings: 4

Ingredients:

10 oz mackerel, chopped

1 white onion, peeled and diced

1 tsp garlic, minced

1/3 cup almond flour

1 egg, beaten

½ tsp thyme

1 tsp salt

1 tsp mustard

1 tsp chili flakes

¼ cup spinach, chopped

4 tbsp coconut oil

Directions:

1. Place mackerel in blender or food processor and blend until texture is smooth.
2. In bowl, combine onion with mackerel.
3. Add garlic, flour, egg, thyme, salt, and mustard, stir well.
4. Add chili flakes and mix up mixture until get homogenous mass.
5. Add spinach and stir.
6. Heat up pan over medium heat and add oil.
7. Shape fish mixture into bombs 1½ inch in diameter.
8. Put bombs on pan and cook for 5 minutes on all sides.
9. Transfer to paper towels and drain grease. Serve.

Nutrition per Serving: Calories - 318, Carbs - 3.45g, Fat – 26.5g, Protein 20.1g

Sardine Fritters

Prep time: 25 minutes | Cook time: 35 minutes | Servings: 6

Ingredients:

2 lbs sardines, minced

1 tsp salt

1 tsp cilantro

½ tbsp ground ginger

¼ cup spinach, chopped roughly

2 tbsp butter

3 tbsp fish stock

4 tbsp coconut milk

Directions:

1. In bowl, combine sardines, salt, cilantro and ginger. Stir gently.
2. Place spinach in blender and blend for 1 minute.
3. Add spinach in sardine mixture and mix well.
4. Shape fish mixture into balls and flatten them.
5. Heat up pan over medium heat and melt butter.
6. Place fish fritters on pan and fry for 2 minutes on one side.
7. Flip on other side; pour in fish stock and coconut milk.
8. Then close lid and simmer fritters for 10 minutes.
9. Serve hot.

Nutrition per Serving: Calories - 369, Carbs - 1g, Fat - 24g, Protein 38g

Grilled Squid with Guacamole

Prep time: 15 minutes | Cook time: 15 minutes | Servings: 3

Ingredients:

2 medium squids

Salt and ground black pepper to taste

½ tsp olive oil

Juice from 1 lime

For the guacamole:

2 avocados, pitted

1 tomato, cored and chopped

Juice from 2 limes

Fresh coriander, chopped

1 onion, peeled and chopped

2 red chilies, chopped

Directions:

1. Separate tentacles from squid and score tubes lengthwise.
2. Rub squid and tentacles with black pepper, salt and olive oil.
3. Heat up grill over medium high heat and put squid and tentacles score side down.
4. Cook for 2 minutes, flip, and cook for 2 minutes more.
5. Transfer to bowl and sprinkle all parts with lime juice.
6. Peel and chop avocado.
7. In medium bowl, mash avocado with fork.
8. Add tomato, juice from 2 limes, coriander, onion, and chilies. Mix well.
9. Serve squid with guacamole.

Nutrition per Serving: Calories - 498, Carbs – 6.95g, Fat – 44.5g, Protein – 19.9g

Fish Meatballs

Prep time: 12 minutes | Cook time: 15 minutes | Servings: 6

Ingredients:

15 oz salmon, chopped roughly

½ tsp chili flakes

1 tsp parsley, chopped

1 tbsp dill, chopped

1 tsp kosher salt

1 tsp garlic, minced

2 eggs, beaten

8 oz almond flour

4 tbsp butter

¼ cup fish stock

Directions:

1. Place salmon in blender or food processor and blend until smooth.
2. In medium bowl, mix together chili flakes, parsley, dill, and salt.
3. Add blended salmon to spice mixture and stir well.
4. Add garlic and eggs, stir carefully until get homogeneous mass.
5. Shape mixture into meatballs 1½ inch in diameter and set aside.
6. Sprinkle meatballs with almond flour.
7. Preheat pan on medium heat and melt butter.
8. Put fish meatballs in pan and cook on high heat for 1 minute on both sides.
9. Then, add fish stock and close lid. Simmer for 10 minutes on medium heat.
10. Serve hot.

Nutrition per Serving: Calories - 209, Carbs - 1.75g, Fat – 16.1g, Protein - 16.8g

Tasty Coconut Cod

Prep time: 30 Minutes | Cook time: 12 Minutes | Servings: 4

Ingredients:

24 oz cod fillets

1½ cups coconut flour

¼ tsp sea salt

1½ tsp ginger powder

1 cup coconut, finely shredded

2 cups coconut milk

2 tbsp coconut oil

Directions:

1. Rinse and debone the fish fillets, then slice into small strips.
2. In medium bowl, mix together coconut flour, salt and ginger.
3. In small bowl add shredded coconut.
4. In another medium bowl, pour in coconut milk.
5. Heat up pan over high heat and add oil.
6. Toss fillets into coconut milk, then into the flour mixture, back into the milk, and finally into shredded coconut.
7. Place on pan and fry for 4-5 minutes per side.
8. Serve fish fillets hot.

Nutrition per Serving: Calories – 599, Carbs – 12.9g, Fat - 45g, Protein – 42.9g

Curry Cod Bites

Prep time: 12 minutes | Cook time: 20 minutes | Servings: 3

Ingredients:

10 oz cod, chopped into 1-inch cubes

1 tsp salt

½ tsp paprika

1 tsp ground ginger

1 tsp curry paste

1 tsp oregano

1 tsp cilantro

½ tsp chili pepper

3 cloves garlic, peeled and sliced

3 eggs, beaten and whisked

2 tbsp butter

2 oz water

Directions:

1. Season fish cubes with salt.
2. In small bowl, mix together paprika, ground ginger, curry paste, oregano, cilantro, and chili pepper.
3. Season fish with spice mixture.
4. Add sliced garlic and stir gently.
5. Add spicy cod to whisked eggs and stir.
6. Heat up pan over medium heat and melt butter.
7. Transfer fish mixture to pan and cook for 10 minutes, stirring constantly.
8. Then increase heat, add water and simmer for another 5 minutes.
9. Serve dish hot.

Nutrition per Serving: Calories - 318, Carbs - 4.44g, Fat – 20.2g, Protein – 8.85g

Trout Stew

Prep time: 15 minutes | Cook time: 30 minutes | Servings: 4

Ingredients:

1 tsp coriander

1 tbsp lemon juice

1 tsp salt

1 tbsp garlic, minced

14 oz trout, chopped roughly

2 cups water

1 cup asparagus, cut in half

1 cup tomatoes, chopped

1 green bell pepper, deseeded and sliced

½ cup white onion, diced

2 tbsp butter

Directions:

1. In bowl, combine coriander, lemon juice, salt and garlic.
2. Rub fish chunks with spice mixture and let marinate for 5-10 minutes.
3. Pour water into saucepan and add trout mixture.
4. Cook on medium heat until start to simmer.
5. Add asparagus, tomatoes and bell pepper and simmer for 5 minutes.
6. Add onion and butter, stir.
7. Close lid and continue to simmer for 10 minutes.
8. Open lid and stir carefully. Serve hot.

Nutrition per Serving: Calories - 220, Carbs – 4.98g, Fat - 12g, Protein – 21.9g

Coconut Soup

Prep time: 15 minutes | Cook time: 35 minutes | Servings: 6

Ingredients:

1½ cups coconut milk

4 cups chicken stock

1 tsp fried lemongrass

3 lime leaves

4 Thai chilies, dried and chopped

1-inch fresh ginger, peeled and grated

1 cup fresh cilantro, chopped

Salt and ground black pepper to taste

1 tbsp fish sauce

1 tbsp coconut oil

2 tbsp mushrooms, chopped

4 oz shrimp, peeled and deveined

2 tbsp onion, chopped

1 tbsp fresh cilantro, chopped

Juice from 1 lime

Directions:

1. In medium pot, combine coconut milk, chicken stock, lemongrass and lime leaves.
2. Preheat pot on medium heat.
3. Add Thai chilies, ginger, cilantro, salt and pepper, stir and bring to simmer. Cook for 20 minutes.
4. Strain soup and return liquid to pot.
5. Heat up soup over medium heat.
6. Add fish sauce, coconut oil, mushrooms, shrimp, and onion. Stir well. Cook for 10 minutes.
7. Add cilantro and lime juice, stir. Set aside for 10 minutes.
8. Serve.

Nutrition per Serving: Calories - 448, Carbs – 7.9g, Fat – 33.8g, Protein – 11.8g

Broccoli Soup

Prep time: 12 minutes | Cook time: 35 minutes | Servings: 4

Ingredients:

2 cloves garlic

1 medium white onion

1 tbsp butter

2 cups water

2 cups vegetable stock

1 cup heavy cream

Salt and ground black pepper to taste

½ tsp paprika

1½ cups broccoli, divided into florets

1 cup cheddar cheese

Directions:

1. Peel and mince garlic. Peel and chop onion.
2. Preheat pot on medium heat, add butter and melt it.
3. Add garlic and onion and sauté for 5 minutes, stirring occasionally.
4. Pour in water, vegetable stock, heavy cream and add pepper, salt and paprika.
5. Stir and bring to boil.
6. Add broccoli and simmer for 25 minutes.
7. After that, transfer soup mixture to food processor and blend well.
8. Grate cheddar cheese and add to food processor, blend again.
9. Serve soup hot.

Nutrition per Serving: Calories - 348, Carbs – 6.8g, Fat – 33.8g, Protein – 10.9g

Simple Tomato Soup

Prep time: 15 minutes | Cook time: 10 minutes | Servings: 6

Ingredients:

4 cups canned tomato soup

2 tbsp apple cider vinegar

1 tsp dried oregano

4 tbsp butter

2 tsp turmeric

2 oz red hot sauce

Salt and ground black pepper to taste

4 tbsp olive oil

8 bacon strips, cooked and crumbled

4 oz fresh basil leaves, chopped

4 oz green onions, chopped

Directions:

1. Pour tomato soup in pot and preheat on medium heat. Bring to boil.
2. Add vinegar, oregano, butter, turmeric, hot sauce, salt, black pepper and olive oil. Stir well.
3. Simmer soup for 5 minutes.
4. Serve soup topped with crumbled bacon, green onion and basil.

Nutrition per Serving: Calories - 397, Carbs – 9.8g, Fat – 33.8, Protein – 11.7g

Green Soup

Prep time: 12 minutes | Cook time: 15 minutes | Servings: 6

Ingredients:

2 cloves garlic

1 white onion

1 cauliflower head

2 oz butter

1 bay leaf, crushed

1 cup spinach leaves

½ cup watercress

4 cups vegetable stock

Salt and ground black pepper to taste

1 cup coconut milk

½ cup parsley, for serving

Directions:

1. Peel and mince garlic. Peel and dice onion.
2. Divide cauliflower into florets.
3. Preheat pot on medium high heat, add butter and melt it.
4. Add onion and garlic, stir and sauté for 4 minutes.
5. Add cauliflower and bay leaf, stir and cook for 5 minutes.
6. Add spinach and watercress, stir and cook for another 3 minutes.
7. Pour in vegetable stock. Season with salt and black pepper. Stir and bring to boil.
8. Pour in coconut milk and stir well. Take off heat.
9. Use an immersion blender to blend well.
10. Top with parsley and serve hot.

Nutrition per Serving: Calories - 227, Carbs – 4.89g, Fat – 35.1, Protein – 6.97g

Sausage and Peppers Soup

Prep time: 15 minutes | Cook time: 1 hour 15 minutes | Servings: 6

Ingredients:

1 tbsp avocado oil

2 lbs pork sausage meat

Salt and ground black pepper to taste

1 green bell pepper, seeded and chopped

5 oz canned jalapeños, chopped

5 oz canned tomatoes, chopped

1¼ cup spinach

4 cups beef stock

1 tsp Italian seasoning

1 tbsp cumin

1 tsp onion powder

1 tsp garlic powder

1 tbsp chili powder

Directions:

1. Preheat pot with avocado oil on medium heat.
2. Put sausage meat in pot and brown for 3 minutes on all sides.
3. Add salt, black pepper and green bell pepper and continue to cook for 3 minutes.
4. Add jalapeños and tomatoes, stir well and cook for 2 minutes more.
5. Toss spinach and stir again, close lid and cook for 7 minutes.
6. Pour in beef stock, Italian seasoning, cumin, onion powder, chili powder, garlic powder, salt and black pepper, stir well. Close lid again. Cook for 30 minutes.
7. When time is up, uncover pot and simmer for 15 minutes more.
8. Serve hot.

Nutrition per Serving: Calories - 531, Carbs – 3.99g, Fat – 44.5g, Protein – 25.8g

Avocado Soup

Prep time: 12 minutes | Cook time: 15 minutes | Servings: 4

Ingredients:

2 tbsp butter

2 scallions, chopped

3 cups chicken stock

2 avocados, pitted, peeled, and chopped

Salt and ground black pepper to taste

⅔ cup heavy cream

Directions:

1. Preheat pot on medium heat, add butter and melt it.
2. Toss scallions, stir and sauté for 2 minutes.
3. Pour in 2 ½ cups stock and bring to simmer. Cook for 3 minutes.
4. Meanwhile, peel and chop avocados.
5. Place avocado, ½ cup of stock, cream, salt and pepper in blender and blend well.
6. Add avocado mixture to pot and mix well. Cook for 2 minutes.
7. Sprinkle with more salt and pepper, stir.
8. Serve hot.

Nutrition per Serving: Calories - 329, Carbs – 5.9g, Fat – 22.9g, Protein – 5.8g

Avocado and Bacon Soup

Prep time: 15 minutes | Cook time: 15 minutes | Servings: 6

Ingredients:

1 quart chicken stock

2 avocados, pitted

⅓ cup fresh cilantro, chopped

1 tsp garlic powder

Salt and ground black pepper to taste

Juice of ½ lime

½ lb bacon, cooked and chopped

Directions:

1. Pour chicken stock in pot and bring to boil over medium high heat.
2. Meanwhile, peeled and chopped avocados.
3. Place avocados, cilantro, garlic powder, salt, black pepper and lime juice in blender or food processor and blend well.
4. Add avocado mixture in boiling stock and stir well.
5. Add bacon and season with salt and pepper to taste.
6. Stir and simmer for 3-4 minutes on medium heat.
7. Serve hot.

Nutrition per Serving: Calories - 298, Carbs – 5.98g, Fat – 22.8g, Protein – 16.8g

Roasted Bell Peppers Soup

Prep time: 15 minutes | Cook time: 20 minutes | Servings: 6

Ingredients:

1 medium white onion

2 cloves garlic

2 celery stalks

12 oz roasted bell peppers, seeded

2 tbsp olive oil

Salt and ground black pepper to taste

1 quart chicken stock

2/3 cup water

¼ cup Parmesan cheese, grated

⅔ cup heavy cream

Directions:

1. Peel and chop onion and garlic. Chop celery and bell pepper.
2. Preheat pot with oil on medium heat.
3. Put garlic, onion, celery, salt and pepper in pot, stir and sauté for 8 minutes.
4. Pour in chicken stock and water. Add bell peppers and stir.
5. Bring to boil, close lid and simmer for 5 minutes. Reduce heat if needed.
6. When time is up, blend soup using immersion blender.
7. Add cream and season with salt and pepper to taste. Take off heat.
8. Serve hot with grated cheese.

Nutrition per Serving: Calories - 180, Carbs – 3.9g, Fat – 12.9g, Protein – 5.9g

Spicy Bacon Soup

Prep time: 15 minutes | Cook time: 30 minutes | Servings: 6

Ingredients:

10 oz bacon, chopped

Salt to taste

1 tbsp olive oil

2/3 cup cauliflower, divided into florets

4 oz green bell pepper, seeded and chopped

1 jalapeno pepper, seeded and chopped

4 cups chicken stock

2 tbsp full-fat cream

1 tsp ground black pepper

1 tsp chili pepper

Directions:

1. In bowl, combine bacon with salt.
2. Heat up pan over medium heat and cook bacon for 5 minutes, stirring constantly.
3. Remove bacon from pan and set aside.
4. Pour olive oil in pan and add cauliflower, bell pepper and jalapeno.
5. Cook veggies on high heat for 1 minute, stirring occasionally.
6. In saucepan, mix bacon with vegetables. Pour in chicken stock. Stir.
7. Close lid and cook for 20-25 minutes.
8. Open lid and add cream, stir.
9. Season with salt, black pepper and chili pepper. Stir and cook for 5 minutes more.
10. Serve.

Nutrition per Serving: Calories - 301, Carbs – 3.9g, Fat - 23g, Protein - 19g

Italian Sausage Soup

Prep time: 15 minutes | Cook time: 35 minutes | Servings: 10

Ingredients:

1 tsp avocado oil

2 cloves garlic

1 medium white onion

1½ lbs hot pork sausage, chopped

8 cups chicken stock

1 lb radishes, chopped

10 oz spinach

1 cup heavy cream

6 bacon slices, chopped

Salt and ground black pepper to taste

A pinch of red pepper flakes

Directions:

1. Preheat pot on medium high heat and add oil.
2. Peel and chop garlic and onion.
3. Put garlic, onion and sausage in pot and stir.
4. Cook for few minutes until browned.
5. Pour in chicken stock; add radishes and spinach, stir.
6. Bring mixture to simmer and add cream, bacon, black pepper, salt and red pepper flakes, stir well.
7. Simmer for 20 minutes.
8. Serve hot.

Nutrition per Serving: Calories - 289, Carbs – 3.8g, Fat – 21.8g, Protein – 18.1g

Cabbage Soup with Chorizo Sausages

Prep time: 20 minutes | Cook time: 25 minutes | Servings: 5

Ingredients:

½ tbsp olive oil

10 oz chorizo sausages, sliced

½ tsp oregano

½ tsp cayenne pepper

1 tsp onion powder

1 tsp cilantro

½ tsp ground black pepper

1 tsp kosher salt

11 oz white cabbage, chopped

1 medium white onion, peeled and diced

5 cloves garlic, peeled and sliced

4 cups water

1 green bell pepper, seeded and diced

Directions:

1. Heat up pan over medium heat and add oil.
2. Add sausages and brown them for 2 minutes, stirring constantly.
3. In medium bowl, mix together oregano, cayenne pepper, onion powder, cilantro, black pepper and salt.
4. In another bowl, combine cabbage, onion, and garlic.
5. Season vegetables with spice mixture and stir.
6. Pour water into saucepan and bring to boil over high heat.
7. Add bell pepper and cabbage mixture.
8. Cook for 10 minutes on medium heat.
9. Add sausages and cook for another 10 minutes on low heat.
10. When time is up, take off heat and leave soup for 5-10 minutes.
11. Serve hot.

Nutrition per Serving: Calories - 299, Carbs – 10.1g, Fat – 23.2g, Protein – 14.9g

Vegetable Stew

Prep time: 17 minutes | Cook time: 30 minutes | Servings: 5

Ingredients:

3 cups chicken stock

5.5 oz eggplants, peeled and chopped

5.5 oz cauliflower, divided into florets

1 tsp kosher salt

1 tsp oregano

1 tsp basil

1 tsp olive oil

¼ cup white onion, peeled and chopped

1 cup green bell pepper, seeded and chopped

3 tbsp butter

½ cup spinach, chopped roughly

Directions:

1. Sprinkle eggplants and cauliflower with salt to get rid of bitterness.
2. In small bowl, combine oregano and basil.
3. Preheat pan with olive oil on medium heat.
4. Add chopped onion and sauté for 2 minutes.
5. Then add eggplants and cook them for 5 minutes, stirring constantly.
6. Add cauliflower and fry for another 2 minutes.
7. Transfer fried veggies to saucepan.
8. Add spice mixture.
9. Add green bell pepper and 2 tablespoon of butter.
10. Pour in stock, close lid and simmer for 10 minutes on medium heat.
11. Heat up pan again over medium heat and add 1 tablespoon of butter, melt it.
12. Toss spinach on pan and cook for 2 minutes.
13. Then add spinach to saucepan with vegetables, stir and cook for 15 minutes more.
14. When time is up, stir and serve hot.

Nutrition per Serving: Calories - 99, Carbs - 7g, Fat - 8.65g, Protein - 2g

Spinach Soup

Prep time: 15 minutes | Cook time: 20 minutes | Servings: 6

Ingredients:

1 medium white onion

2½ cups spinach

2 tbsp butter

1 tsp garlic, minced

5½ cups chicken stock

2 cups heavy cream

½ tsp ground nutmeg

Salt and ground black pepper to taste

Directions:

1. Peel and chop onion. Chop spinach.
2. Preheat pot with butter on medium heat.
3. Add onion and sauté for 4 minutes, stirring frequently.
4. Toss garlic, stir and sauté for 1 minute more.
5. Pour in chicken stock and add spinach, stir and cook for 5 minutes.
6. With immersion blender, blend soup well.
7. Heat up soup again; add cream, nutmeg, pepper and salt.
8. Simmer for 5 minutes.
9. Serve hot.

Nutrition per Serving: Calories - 239, Carbs – 3.98g, Fat – 23.9g, Protein – 5.98g

Salads

Lunch Caesar Salad

Prep time: 15 minutes | Cook time: 0 minutes | Servings: 2

Ingredients:

1 avocado, pitted

1 chicken breast, grilled and shredded

1 cup bacon, cooked and crumbled

3 tbsp creamy Caesar dressing

Salt and ground black pepper to taste

Directions:

1. Peel and slice avocado.
2. In medium bowl, combine bacon, chicken breast and avocado.
3. Add creamy Cesar dressing, stir well.
4. Season with salt and pepper, stir.
5. Serve.

Nutrition per Serving: Calories - 329, Carbs – 2.99g, Fat – 22.9g, Protein – 17.8g

Asian Side Salad

Prep time: 35 minutes | Cook time: 12 minutes | Servings: 4

Ingredients:

1 green onion

1 cucumber

2 tbsp coconut oil

1 packet Asian noodles, cooked

¼ tsp red pepper flakes

1 tbsp sesame oil

1 tbsp balsamic vinegar

1 tsp sesame seeds

Salt and ground black pepper to taste

Directions:

1. Chop onion. Slice cucumber thin.
2. Preheat pan with oil on medium high heat.
3. Add cooked noodles and close lid.
4. Fry noodles for 5 minutes until crispy.
5. Transfer noodles to paper towels and drain grease.
6. Combine cucumber, pepper flakes, green onion, sesame oil, vinegar, sesame seeds, pepper, salt and noodles. Mix well.
7. Put in refrigerator at least for 20-30 minutes. Serve.

Nutrition per Serving: Calories - 397, Carbs – 3.97g, Fat – 33.7g, Protein – 1.98g

Keto Egg Salad

Prep time: 15 minutes | Cook time: 0 minutes | Servings: 4

Ingredients:

6 oz ham, chopped

5 eggs, boiled and chopped

1 tsp garlic, minced

½ tsp basil

1 tsp oregano

1 tbsp apple cider vinegar

1 tsp kosher salt

½ cup cream cheese

Directions:

1. In medium bowl, combine chopped ham with chopped eggs, stir.
2. In another bowl, mix together garlic, basil, oregano, vinegar, and salt. Stir the mixture till you get homogeneous consistency.
3. Whisk together spice mixture and cream cheese.
4. Add cream cheese sauce to egg mixture and stir gently.
5. Serve.

Nutrition per Serving: Calories - 341, Carbs – 4.99g, Fat - 26g, Protein – 22.1g

Cobb Salad

Prep time: 20 minutes | Cook time: 27 minutes | Servings: 1

Ingredients:

1 tbsp olive oil

4 oz chicken breast

2 strips bacon

1 cup spinach, chopped roughly

1 large hard-boiled egg, peeled and chopped

¼ avocado, peeled and chopped

½ tsp white vinegar

Directions:

1. Heat up pan on medium heat and add oil.
2. Add chicken breast and bacon, cook until get desired crispiness.
3. Add spinach and egg, stir.
4. Add avocado and mix well.
5. Sprinkle with white vinegar and stir.
6. Serve.

Nutrition per Serving: Calories - 589, Carbs – 2g, Fat – 47.8g, Protein – 42g

Bacon and Zucchini Noodles Salad

Prep time: 15 minutes | Cook time: 0 minutes | Servings: 3

Ingredients:

32 oz zucchini noodles

1 cup baby spinach

⅓ cup blue cheese, crumbled

½ cup bacon, cooked and crumbled

⅓ cup blue cheese dressing

Ground black pepper to taste

Directions:

1. Combine zucchini noodles, spinach, blue cheese, and bacon, Stir carefully.
2. Add black pepper and cheese dressing, toss to coat. Serve.

Nutrition per Serving: Calories - 198, Carbs – 1.99g, Fat – 13.9g, Protein – 9.95g

Chicken Salad

Prep time: 15 minutes | Cook time: 0 minutes | Servings: 3

Ingredients:

1 celery stalk

2 tbsp fresh parsley

1 green onion

5 oz chicken breast, roasted and chopped

1 egg, hard-boiled, peeled and chopped

Salt and ground black pepper to taste

½ tsp garlic powder

⅓ cup mayonnaise

1 tsp mustard

½ tbsp dill relish

Directions:

1. Wash and chop celery, parsley and onion.
2. Place celery, onion and parsley in blender or food processor and blend well.
3. Remove this mass from food processor and set aside.
4. Place chicken in food processor and pulse well.
5. Add chicken to onion mixture and stir.
6. Add egg, pepper and salt, stir gently.
7. Add garlic powder, mayonnaise, mustard and dill relish, toss to coat.
8. Serve.

Nutrition per Serving: Calories - 279, Carbs – 2.99g, Fat – 22.9g, Protein – 11.9g

Asparagus Salad

Prep time: 20 minutes | Cook time: 0 minutes | Servings: 5

Ingredients:

2 lbs asparagus, cooked and halved

1 tbsp butter, melted

½ tsp garlic powder

1 tsp sesame seeds

1 tbsp coconut oil

1 tbsp apple cider vinegar

1 tsp dried basil

1 tsp salt

4 oz Parmesan cheese, grated

Directions:

1. In bowl, combine asparagus, butter and garlic powder. Stir well.
2. Add sesame seeds, coconut oil, vinegar, basil and salt. Mix well.
3. Set salad aside to marinate.
4. Serve salad with grated Parmesan cheese.

Nutrition per Serving: Calories - 133, Carbs - 7g, Fat - 8.85g, Protein - 10g

Apple Salad

Prep time: 15 minutes | Cook time: 0 minutes | Servings: 4

Ingredients:

1 medium apple

2 oz pecans

16 oz broccoli florets

1 green onion

2 tsp poppy seeds

Salt and ground black pepper to taste

¼ cup sour cream

¼ cup mayonnaise

½ tsp lemon juice

1 tsp apple cider vinegar

Directions:

1. Core and grate apple. Chop pecans and broccoli florets. Dice green onion.
2. In bowl, combine broccoli, apple, pecans, and green onion. Stir well.
3. Sprinkle with poppy seeds, black pepper and salt, stir carefully.
4. In another bowl, whisk sour cream, mayonnaise, lemon juice and vinegar.
5. Add this mixture to salad and toss to coat.
6. Serve.

Nutrition per Serving: Calories - 249, Carbs – 3.9g, Fat – 22.9g, Protein – 4.8g

Bok Choy Salad

Prep time: 20 minutes | Cook time: 10 minutes | Servings: 6

Ingredients:

10 oz bok choy, chopped roughly

2 tbsp coconut oil

4 tbsp chicken stock

1 tsp basil

1 tsp ground black pepper

1 white onion, peeled and sliced

¼ cup white mushrooms, marinated and chopped

1 lb tofu, chopped

1 tsp oregano

1 tsp almond milk

Directions:
1. Heat up pan on medium heat.
2. Add bok choy, 1 tablespoon of oil and chicken stock.
3. Season with basil and black pepper.
4. Add onion and close lid.
5. Simmer vegetables for 5-6 minutes, stirring constantly.
6. Transfer vegetables to bowl and add mushrooms.
7. Pour 1 tablespoon of oil in pan and heat it up again.
8. Add chopped tofu and cook for 2 minutes.
9. Transfer tofu to bowl with vegetables and sprinkle with oregano.
10. Pour in almond milk and toss to coat.
11. Serve salad.

Nutrition per Serving: Calories - 130, Carbs - 4.67g, Fat - 11g, Protein – 6.9g

Halloumi Salad

Prep time: 15 minutes | Cook time: 12 minutes | Servings: 2

Ingredients:

3 oz halloumi cheese, sliced

1 cucumber, sliced

½ cup baby arugula

5 cherry tomatoes, halved

1 oz walnuts, chopped

Salt and ground black pepper to taste

½ tsp olive oil

¼ tsp balsamic vinegar

Directions:

1. Preheat grill on medium high heat.
2. Put halloumi cheese in grill and cook for 5 minutes per side.
3. In mixing bowl, combine cucumber, arugula, tomatoes, and walnuts.
4. Place halloumi pieces on top.
5. Sprinkle with black pepper and salt.
6. Drizzle oil and balsamic vinegar, toss to coat.
7. Serve.

Nutrition per Serving: Calories - 448, Carbs – 3.98g, Fat – 42.8g, Protein – 22.3g

Smoked Salmon Salad

Prep time: 17 minutes | Cook time: 0 minutes | Servings: 4

Ingredients:

8 oz smoked salmon, sliced into thin pieces

2 oz pecans, crushed

3 medium tomatoes, chopped

½ cup lettuce, chopped

1 cucumber, diced

1/3 cup cream cheese

1/3 cup coconut milk

½ tsp oregano

1 tbsp lemon juice, chopped

½ tsp basil

1 tsp salt

Directions:

1. In medium bowl, combine salmon with pecans and stir.
2. Add tomatoes, lettuce and cucumber, stir well.
3. In another bowl, mix together cream cheese, coconut milk, oregano, lemon juice, basil and salt. Stir mixture until get homogenous mass.
4. Serve salmon salad with cream cheese sauce.

Nutrition per Serving: Calories - 211, Carbs – 7.1g, Fat – 15.9g, Protein – 9.95g

Tuna Salad

Prep time: 18 minutes | Cook time: 0 minutes | Servings: 4

Ingredients:

1 can tuna

4 eggs, boiled, peeled and chopped

1 oz olives, pitted and sliced

1/3 cup cheese cream

½ cup almond milk

½ tsp ground black pepper

½ tsp kosher salt

1 tbsp garlic, minced

Directions:

1. In medium bowl, mash tuna with fork.
2. Add chopped eggs and stir.
3. Add sliced olives and stir.
4. In another bowl, whisk together cheese cream and almond milk.
5. Add black pepper, salt and garlic, stir carefully.
6. Add cheese mixture to tuna mixture and mix up.
7. Serve.

Nutrition per Serving: Calories - 182, Carbs - 8g, Fat – 11.9g, Protein - 12.88g

Caprese Salad

Prep time: 7 minutes | Cook time: 0 minutes | Servings: 2

Ingredients:

8 oz mozzarella cheese

1 medium tomato

4 basil leaves

Salt and ground black pepper to taste

3 tsp balsamic vinegar

1 tbsp olive oil

Directions:

1. Slice mozzarella cheese and tomato. Torn basil leaves.
2. Alternate tomato and mozzarella slices on 2 plates.
3. Season with pepper and salt.
4. Drizzle vinegar and olive oil.
5. Sprinkle with the basil leaves.
6. Serve.

Nutrition per Serving: Calories - 148, Carbs – 5.9g, Fat – 11.8g, Protein – 8.95g

Warm Bacon Salad

Prep time: 16 minutes | Cook time: 18 minutes | Servings: 5

Ingredients:

16 oz bacon strips, chopped

1 tsp cilantro

1 tsp ground ginger

1 tsp kosher salt

2 tbsp butter

3 boiled eggs, peeled and chopped

2 tomatoes, diced

1 oz spinach, chopped

4 oz Cheddar cheese, grated

1 tsp almond milk

7 oz eggplant, peeled and diced

Directions:

1. In medium bowl, combine bacon, cilantro, ginger and salt.
2. Heat up pan over medium heat and melt 1 tablespoon of butter.
3. Put bacon in pan and cook for 5 minutes. Transfer bacon to plate.
4. Meanwhile, in bowl, mix together chopped eggs, tomatoes and spinach.
5. Sprinkle with cheese and add almond milk.
6. Heat up pan again over medium heat and melt remaining 1 tablespoon of butter.
7. Add diced eggplants and fry for 8 minutes, stirring occasionally.
8. Then add bacon and roasted eggplants to salad.
9. Season with salt and stir gently.
10. Serve.

Nutrition per Serving: Calories - 159, Carbs - 4.22g, Fat - 13g, Protein - 8.75g

Cauliflower Side Salad

Prep time: 14 minutes | Cook time: 7 minutes | Servings: 8

Ingredients:

21 oz cauliflower

1 tbsp water

4 boiled eggs, peeled and chopped

1 cup onion, chopped

1 cup celery, chopped

1 cup mayonnaise

Salt and ground black pepper to taste

2 tbsp cider vinegar

1 tsp sucralose

Directions:

1. Divide cauliflower into florets and put them in heatproof bowl.
2. Add water and place in microwave, cook for 5 minutes.
3. Transfer to serving bowl.
4. Add eggs, onions, and celery. Stir gently.
5. In another bowl, whisk together mayonnaise, black pepper, salt, vinegar and sucralose.
6. Add this sauce to salad and toss to coat.
7. Serve.

Nutrition per Serving: Calories - 209, Carbs – 2.9g, Fat – 19.7g, Protein – 3.97g

Keto Tricolor Salad

Prep time: 12 minutes | Cook time: 8 minutes | Servings: 5

Ingredients:

5 oz mozzarella cheese

1 tsp oregano

1 tsp minced garlic

1 tsp basil

1 tbsp coconut oil

1 tsp lemon juice

2 medium tomatoes, sliced

7 oz avocado, pitted and sliced

8 olives, pitted and sliced

Directions:

1. Cut mozzarella cheese balls into halves.
2. In medium bowl, mix together oregano, garlic, basil, coconut oil and lemon juice.
3. On serving plate place sliced tomato, then place sliced avocado and olives.
4. Put mozzarella pieces on top.
5. Drizzle coconut sauce over salad and serve.

Nutrition per Serving: Calories - 239, Carbs – 7.9g, Fat – 20.1g, Protein - 11.77g

Shrimp Salad with Grapefruit and Avocado

Prep Time: 15 Minutes | Cook Time: 12 Minutes | Servings: 2

Ingredients:

2 tbsp chili oil

1 cup shrimp, peeled

½ tsp pepper

½ tsp salt

1 avocado, peeled and cubed

1 grapefruit, peeled and cubed

2 oz lemon juice

Directions:

1. Preheat saucepan with chili oil on medium heat.
2. Add shrimp and fry until opaque and lightly brown.
3. Transfer shrimp to bowl and sprinkle with salt and pepper.
4. In serving bowl, layer avocado cubes as tightly as possible, then layer shrimp, and top with grapefruit.
5. Drizzle with lemon juice.
6. Serve immediately.

Nutrition per Serving: Calories – 492, Carbs - 17g, Fat – 36.1g, Protein – 27.9g

Greek Salad

Prep time: 15 minutes | Cook time: 7 minutes | Servings: 3

Ingredients:

1 cucumber, chopped

2 tomatoes, chopped

6 oz Parmesan cheese, cut into cubes

1 white onion, peeled and sliced

3 oz black olives, pitted and halved

1 tsp oregano

1 tsp kosher salt

½ tsp ground black pepper

1 tsp salt

1 tsp basil

1 tbsp coconut oil

Directions:

1. In medium bowl, combine cucumber, tomatoes, Parmesan cheese and onion. Stir carefully.
2. Add olives and stir.
3. Season with oregano, salt, black pepper, basil and coconut oil. Stir gently.
4. Serve

Nutrition per Serving: Calories – 299, Carbs - 12g, Fat – 19.9g, Protein – 19.9g

Vegetable Frittata

Prep time: 25 minutes | Cook time: 28 minutes |Servings: 6

Ingredients:

8 eggs, beaten

1/3 cup almond milk

1 tbsp cilantro

½ tsp turmeric

1 tsp salt

1/3 cup kale, chopped

1 white onion, peeled and diced

1 green bell pepper, chopped

1 cup spinach, chopped

½ cup tomatoes, chopped

4 tbsp butter

Directions:

1. In medium bowl, whisk together eggs, almond milk, cilantro, turmeric, and salt.
2. Add kale, onion and bell pepper, stir.
3. Add spinach and tomatoes, stir carefully.
4. Preheat oven to 370 F.
5. Grease bake form with butter and pour in egg mixture.
6. Place bake form in oven and bake for about 25 minutes.
7. Serve warm.

Nutrition per Serving: Calories - 237, Carbs -5.9g, Fat: 21g, Protein – 9.98g

Spinach Rolls

Prep time: 25 minutes | Cook time: 18 minutes | Servings: 14

Ingredients:

2½ cups mozzarella cheese, shredded

2 eggs, beaten

½ cup almond flour

¼ tsp salt

6 tbsp coconut flour

For the filling:

½ tsp avocado oil

2/3 cup spinach, torn

4 oz cream cheese

¼ cup Parmesan cheese, grated

¼ tsp salt

Mayonnaise, for serving

Directions:

1. Preheat pan on medium heat and add oil.
2. Toss spinach on pan and cook for 2 minutes.
3. Add cream cheese, Parmesan cheese, and salt. Mix well and take off heat, leave aside.
4. Place mozzarella in heatproof bowl and put in microwave for 30 seconds.
5. Add eggs, almond flour, salt and coconut flour, mix well.
6. Flatten dough with rolling pin on lined cutting board.
7. Divide the dough into 14-16 rectangles.
8. Spread spinach mixture on each rectangle and roll them into cigar shapes.
9. Preheat oven to 350 F.
10. Put all rolls on baking sheet and place in oven. Cook for 15 minutes.
11. Let rolls chill little and top with some mayonnaise. Serve.

Nutrition per Serving: Calories - 495, Carbs – 13.8g, Fat – 67g, Protein – 33g

Bok Choy Muffins

Prep time: 25 minutes | Cook time: 35 minutes | Servings: 4

Ingredients:

½ medium white onion, diced

2 cup bok choy, chopped into tiny pieces

1 tbsp coconut oil

3 eggs, beaten

½ cup coconut milk

½ cup almond flour

½ tsp baking soda

1 tbsp minced garlic

1 tsp apple cider vinegar

1 tsp salt

3 tbsp butter

Directions:

1. In bowl, mix together onion and bok choy.
2. Heat up skillet with oil on medium heat.
3. Add onion mixture and cook for 5 minutes, stirring constantly.
4. In medium bowl, whisk together eggs and coconut milk.
5. Add almond flour, baking soda, garlic, vinegar, and salt. Stir mixture until smooth.
6. Add onion mixture and mix up dough until get homogeneous consistency.
7. Grease muffin forms with butter and fill ½ of every form with dough.
8. Set oven to 365 F and heat it up.
9. Place muffins in oven and bake for 20 minutes.
10. Let muffins cool down for few minutes and remove from forms. Serve.

Nutrition per Serving: Calories - 275, Carbs - 6,45g, Fat – 25.9g, Protein – 6.9g

Avocado Fries

Prep time: 12 minutes | Cook time: 7 minutes | Servings: 3

Ingredients:

3 avocados, pitted

1½ cups almond meal

¼ tsp cayenne pepper

Salt and ground black pepper to taste

2 eggs, beaten

1½ cups sunflower oil

Directions:

1. Peel and cut in half avocados, slice it.
2. Combine almond meal, cayenne pepper, black pepper and salt.
3. In another bowl, whisk eggs with salt and black pepper.
4. Preheat pan with oil on medium high heat.
5. Dip avocado slices in egg mixture, then in almond meal mixture and put in pan.
6. Fry slices until they are golden.
7. Transfer to plate with paper towels and drain excess grease. Serve.

Nutrition per Serving: Calories - 448, Carbs – 6.9g, Fat – 44g, Protein – 16.8g

Garlic Mushrooms

Prep time: 17 minutes | Cook time: 22 minutes | Servings: 3

Ingredients:

5 tbsp butter

1 tsp cilantro

2 tbsp minced garlic

½ tsp basil

1 tbsp oregano

1 tsp paprika

8 oz white mushrooms, washed and chopped

Directions:

1. In bowl, mix together butter, cilantro, garlic, basil, oregano and paprika.
2. Put mushrooms in baking form.
3. Add butter mixture and stir gently. Cover form tightly with aluminum foil.
4. Set oven to 360 F and heat it up.
5. Place dish in oven and bake for 20 minutes.
6. Remove foil and bake for another 2 minutes, until mushrooms are soft.
7. Serve hot.

Nutrition per Serving: Calories - 298, Carbs – 7.9g, Fat - 22g, Protein - 5g

Fried Asparagus

Prep Time: 12 Minutes | Cook Time: 12 Minutes | Servings: 6

Ingredients:

2 egg yolks

1 tbsp lemon juice

¼ cup butter

Salt and ground black pepper to taste

A pinch of cayenne pepper

40 asparagus spears

Directions:

1. Whisk egg yolks with lemon juice well.
2. Preheat pan on low heat and pour in egg yolks mixture.
3. Add butter and stir until it melts.
4. Season with black pepper, cayenne pepper and salt, stir.
5. Increase temperature on medium high heat, add asparagus and cook for 5 minutes.
6. Serve warm.

Nutrition per Serving: Calories - 149, Carbs – 1.9g, Fat – 12.9g, Protein – 2.8g

Vegetable lasagna

Prep time: 17 minutes | Cook time: 28 minutes |Servings: 6

Ingredients:

15 oz eggplants, sliced

1 tsp salt

1 tsp paprika

1 tbsp coconut oil

1 cup spinach, chopped roughly

1 cup Cheddar cheese, grated

1 cup Parmesan cheese, grated

1 tsp rosemary

1 tsp ground black pepper

1 tsp chili pepper

7 eggs, beaten

3 tbsp butter

1 tsp minced garlic

1/3 cup cream

Directions:

1. In bowl, season eggplants with salt and paprika.
2. Then sprinkle with coconut oil.
3. Set oven to 365 F and heat it up.
4. Place eggplants in tray and transfer to oven, bake for 10 minutes.
5. Steam spinach: place in microwave safe bowl and cover. Heat in microwave for 2-3 minutes.
6. In medium bowl, combine Cheddar and Parmesan cheese. Season with rosemary, black pepper and chili pepper, stir.
7. Get eggplants out of oven.
8. In another bowl, whisk eggs. Make crepes from whisked egg mixture.
9. Grease baking dish with butter.
10. Make layer of eggplants in dish.
11. Add layer of steamed spinach and sprinkle with cheese mixture.
12. Add egg crepe.
13. Repeat same 3 times.
14. In small bowl, mix together garlic and cream. Stir until get homogenous mass.
15. Pour mixture over lasagna in baking dish.
16. Place dish in oven and cook at 365F for 15 minutes.
17. Serve hot.

Nutrition per Serving: Calories - 451, Carbs – 7.85g, Fat - 35g, Protein – 28.9g

Vegetable Stew

Prep time: 20 minutes | Cook time: 30 minutes | Servings: 5

Ingredients:

5.5 oz eggplants, peeled and chopped

5.5 oz cauliflower, divided into florets

1 tsp salt

1 tsp oregano

1 tsp basil

1 tsp olive oil

1 cup green bell peppers, seeded and chopped roughly

3 tbsp butter

3 cups chicken stock

½ cup spinach, chopped

¼ cup medium white onion, chopped

Directions:

1. In medium bowl, season eggplants and cauliflower florets with salt to get rid of bitterness.
2. In small bowl, combine oregano and basil.
3. Preheat pan with olive oil on medium heat. Add eggplants and fry for 5 minutes, stirring constantly.
4. Add cauliflower and cook for another 2 minutes.
5. Transfer eggplants mixture to saucepan; add bell pepper, 2 tablespoons of butter, and chicken stock. Stir.
6. Cover and simmer for 10 minutes on medium heat.
7. Heat up pan over medium heat again and melt 1 tablespoon of butter.
8. Toss spinach and onion in pan and cook for 2 minutes
9. Transfer spinach to saucepan with stew, stir and cook for 15 minutes more.
10. Serve warm.

Nutrition per Serving: Calories - 110, Carbs - 7g, Fat - 8.55g, Protein - 2g

Broccoli with Lemon Almond Butter

Prep time: 15 minutes | Cook time: 8 minutes | Servings: 4

Ingredients:

¼ cup coconut butter, melted

¼ cup almonds, blanched

2 tbsp lemon juice

1 tsp lemon zest

1 broccoli head, divided into florets and steamed

Salt and ground black pepper to taste

Directions:

1. Preheat pan on medium heat and add coconut butter.
2. Add almonds, lemon juice and lemon zest, stir until butter melts. Take off heat.
3. Add broccoli to pan and toss to coat. Season with salt and pepper.
4. Serve.

Nutrition per Serving: Calories - 168, Carbs – 3.98g, Fat – 14.9g, Protein – 3.9g

Broccoli Croquets

Prep time: 20 minutes | Cook time: 12 minutes | Servings: 4

Ingredients:

10 oz broccoli, chopped roughly

1 tsp onion powder

1 tsp turmeric

1 tsp salt

1 tsp paprika

3 eggs, beaten

1 tbsp flax meal

1 cup spinach, chopped into tiny pieces

½ cup coconut flour

6 oz bacon, chopped

4 tbsp butter

Directions:

1. Place broccoli in blender or food processor and blend until smooth.
2. Transfer this mass to bowl and add onion powder, turmeric, salt, and paprika. Stir.
3. Add eggs in bowl and mix until get homogenous mass.
4. Add flax meal and stir.
5. Add spinach to bowl and mix well.
6. Add coconut flour and bacon, stir carefully.
7. Heat up pan on medium heat and melt butter.
8. Shape mixture into croquets 1½-2 inch in diameter and put in pan.
9. Cook for 4 minutes on both sides.
10. Serve warm.

Nutrition per Serving: Calories - 293, Carbs - 6,45g, Fat – 23.1g, Protein - 15,68g

Kale Paste

Prep time: 25 minutes | Cook time: 35 minutes | Servings: 4

Ingredients:

8 oz spinach, chopped roughly

8 oz kale, chopped roughly

3 tbsp butter

½ cup almond milk

1 tsp ground black pepper

1 tsp turmeric

1 tsp oregano

1 tbsp almond flour

3 tbsp Parmesan cheese, grated

Directions:

1. Place spinach and kale in blender or food processor and blend for about 3 minutes until get smooth consistency.
2. Heat up pan over medium heat and melt butter.
3. Put vegetable mixture in pan.
4. Pour in almond milk and season with black pepper, oregano and turmeric.
5. Add almond flour and stir gently. Close lid.
6. Simmer dish for 7 minutes.
7. After that, add cheese and stir carefully. Simmer for 3 minutes more.
8. Let dish cool down for few minutes and serve.

Nutrition per Serving: Calories - 271, Carbs – 7.1g, Fat – 24.2g, Protein – 10g

Sautéed Broccoli

Prep time: 12 minutes | Cook time: 25 minutes | Servings: 3

Ingredients:

1 clove garlic

5 tbsp olive oil

1 lb broccoli florets, steamed

Salt and ground black pepper to taste

1 tbsp Parmesan cheese

Directions:

1. Peel and mince garlic. Grate Parmesan cheese.
2. Preheat pan with oil on medium high heat.
3. Add minced garlic and sauté for 2 minutes.
4. Add steamed broccoli to pan and cook for 15 minutes, stirring occasionally.
5. Season with salt and pepper, stir carefully.
6. Serve topped with Parmesan cheese.

Nutrition per Serving: Calories - 189, Carbs – 5.94g, Fat – 13.85g, Protein – 4.97g

Cauliflower in Aromatic Batter

Prep time: 12 minutes | Cook time: 23 minutes | Servings: 4

Ingredients:

4 eggs, beaten

½ cup almond milk

1 tsp salt

1 tsp ground black pepper

½ cup almond flour

1 tsp minced garlic

1 tbsp butter

14 oz cauliflower, divided into medium florets

Directions:

1. In bowl, whisk together eggs, almond milk, salt, black pepper, and almond flour.
2. Mix up mixture until smooth.
3. Add garlic and stir.
4. Grease baking dish with butter and put cauliflower florets in it.
5. Pour egg mixture over cauliflower and stir.
6. Set oven to 365 F and heat it up.
7. Place baking dish in oven and bake for 20 minutes.
8. When time is up, let dish cool down for 3-5 minutes.
9. Serve hot.

Nutrition per Serving: Calories - 230, Carbs – 8.45g, Fat – 17.9g, Protein - 10g

Chopped Cabbage Stew

Prep time: 22 minutes | Cook time: 35 minutes | Servings: 8

Ingredients:

1 lb beef brisket, cut into 1½ inch cubes

1 tbsp kosher salt

1 tsp turmeric

1 tsp paprika

1/3 cup cream

2 cups chicken stock

2 jalapeno pepper, seeded and chopped

4 oz red cabbage, chopped

2 lbs white cabbage, chopped

5 celery stalks, chopped

2 white onions, peeled and sliced

Directions:

1. Mix beef cubes with salt, turmeric and paprika.
2. Put meat in saucepan, add cream and chicken stock.
3. Close lid, heat up saucepan over medium heat and simmer dish for 20 minutes.
4. Meanwhile, combine jalapeno pepper, cabbage and celery.
5. Add onion to saucepan, stir and simmer for 5 minutes more.
6. Add cabbage mixture to saucepan, stir and simmer for another 15 minutes on low heat.
7. Let dish cool down for few minutes and serve.

Nutrition per Serving: Calories - 131, Carbs - 6.44g, Fat – 35.9g, Protein - 15.9g

Fried Swiss Chard

Prep time: 15 minutes | Cook time: 12 minutes | Servings: 3

Ingredients:

4 bacon slices

1 bunch Swiss chard

2 tbsp butter

3 tbsp lemon juice

½ tsp garlic paste

Salt and ground black pepper to taste

Directions:

1. Chop bacon slices. Chop Swiss chard.
2. Preheat pan on medium heat. Add chopped bacon and fry until crispy.
3. Toss butter in pan and stir until melts.
4. Add lemon juice and garlic paste, stir. Cook for 1 minute more.
5. Add Swiss chard and stir. Cook for another 4 minutes.
6. Season dish with salt and pepper, stir.
7. Serve hot.

Nutrition per Serving: Calories - 297, Carbs – 5.89g, Fat – 31.8g, Protein – 7.92g

Keto Broccoli Stew

Prep time: 12 minutes | Cook time: 25 minutes | Servings: 4

Ingredients:

1 cup bok choy, chopped roughly

1 cup broccoli, chopped roughly

1 tsp kosher salt

1 tsp paprika

½ quart bone broth

5 oz bacon strips

½ tsp ground black pepper

1 tsp olive oil

¼ cup cream cheese

1 tbsp cream

¼ cup almond milk

Directions:

1. In medium bowl, combine bok choy, broccoli, salt and paprika.
2. Pour bone broth in saucepan.
3. Add vegetable mixture and start to cook on low heat.
4. Season bacon strips with black pepper.
5. Heat up pan with oil over medium heat. Add bacon and cook for 2 minutes.
6. Transfer bacon to saucepan. Stir carefully.
7. In bowl, mix together cream cheese and cream.
8. Add cream mass and almond milk to saucepan. Stir gently.
9. Close lid. Continue simmer stew for 10 minutes.
10. Let stew cool down for few minutes.
11. Serve hot.

Nutrition per Serving: Calories - 211, Carbs - 5g, Fat - 16.84g, Protein - 11.45g

Tasty Broccoli Mash

Prep time: 12 minutes | Cook time: 18 minutes | Servings: 4

Ingredients:

1 cup water

14 oz broccoli, chopped roughly

1 tsp kosher salt

¼ cup coconut milk

2 tbsp butter

3 oz Parmesan cheese, grated

1 oz olives, pitted and sliced

Directions:

1. Pour water in saucepan. Add broccoli and ½ teaspoon salt.
2. Cover and cook broccoli for 10 minutes on medium heat.
3. In medium bowl, whisk together coconut milk, butter and ½ teaspoon salt.
4. When broccoli is cooked, place it in blender or food processor and blend until smooth.
5. Add butter mixture in broccoli and stir.
6. Add cheese and olives in broccoli mixture.
7. Mix up until get homogenous consistency.
8. Serve.

Nutrition per Serving: Calories - 128, Carbs - 5.85g, Fat - 11g, Protein - 6.9g

Twice-Baked Zucchini

Prep time: 12 minutes | Cook time: 35 minutes | Servings: 4

Ingredients:

2 zucchini

2 tbsp butter

1 tbsp jalapeño pepper, seeded and chopped

2 oz onion, peeled and chopped

4 bacon strips, cooked and crumbled

2 oz cream cheese, softened

4 oz cheddar cheese, shredded

¼ cup sour cream

Salt and ground black pepper to taste

Directions:

1. Cut zucchini into half and each half in half lengthwise.
2. Scoop out flesh and put in bowl. Place zucchini cups in baking dish.
3. In mixing bowl, combine zucchini flesh, butter, jalapeño pepper, onion, bacon, cream cheese, cheddar cheese, sour cream, salt and pepper. Mix well.
4. Set oven to 350 F and heat it up.
5. Spread this mixture in zucchini quarters and place baking dish in oven.
6. Bake for 30 minutes. Serve.

Nutrition per Serving: Calories - 258, Carbs – 2.98g, Fat – 21.9g, Protein – 9.9g

Zucchini Wraps with the Cream Cheese

Prep time: 15 minutes | Cook time: 5 minutes | Servings: 4

Ingredients:

1 zucchini, washed and sliced

1 tsp paprika

½ tsp ground black pepper

2 tbsp coconut oil

1/3 cup cream cheese

1 tbsp minced garlic

7 oz Parmesan cheese, grated

Directions:

1. In bowl, mix together zucchini, paprika and black pepper.
2. Heat up pan with coconut oil over medium heat.
3. Fry zucchini for 30 seconds on each side.
4. Transfer zucchini slices to paper towels and drain grease.
5. In bowl, combine garlic with cream cheese. Mix up until get homogenous mass.
6. Add Parmesan cheese and stir carefully.
7. Grease zucchini slices with cream cheese mixture and wrap rolls.
8. Serve.

Nutrition per Serving: Calories - 301, Carbs – 4.98g, Fat - 25g, Protein – 17.9g

Cheddar and Ham Wraps

Prep time: 10 minutes | Cook time: 7 minutes | Servings: 1

Ingredients:

2 tbsp mayonnaise

1 low carb wrap

2 oz cheddar, shredded

2 oz deli ham, slices

Pickles or jalapenos to taste, sliced

Salt and ground black pepper to taste

Directions:

1. Spread mayonnaise on low carb wrap.
2. Sprinkle with shredded cheese.
3. Add ham slices.
4. Add jalapenos or pickles to taste.
5. Sprinkle with salt and black pepper to tasty.
6. Wrap it up and serve.

Nutrition per Serving: Calories - 595, Carbs – 7.9g, Fat – 43.7g, Protein – 26.8g

Easy Avocado Wraps

Prep time: 10 minutes | Cook time: 0 minutes | Servings: 1

Ingredients:
3 lettuce leaves

3 tbsp mayonnaise

6 strips bacon, cooked

½ roma tomato, sliced

½ avocado, sliced

Salt and ground black pepper to taste

Directions:
1. Carefully flatten lettuce leaves and add tablespoon of mayonnaise to each.
2. Then put 2 bacon strips on each leaf.
3. Then place tomato and avocado on top.
4. Sprinkle with salt and black pepper.
5. Wrap each leaf tightly. Serve.

Nutrition per Serving: Calories - 633, Carbs – 5.9g, Fat – 55.5g, Protein – 17.8g

Crispy Zucchini Circles with Parmesan Cheese

Prep time: 25 minutes | Cook time: 33 minutes | Servings: 4

Ingredients:

2 zucchini, washed and sliced

1 tsp basil

½ tsp cilantro

7 oz Cheddar cheese, grated

6 oz Parmesan cheese, grated

1 tbsp butter

½ tbsp minced garlic

1 tbsp coconut oil

Directions:

1. In medium bowl, combine zucchini slices, basil and cilantro.
2. In another bowl, mix together Cheddar cheese, Parmesan cheese, garlic and butter.
3. Set oven to 370 F and heat it up.
4. Cover the tray with the baking paper and transfer the sliced zucchini in the tray.
5. Season zucchini slices with cheese mixture and spray with coconut oil.
6. Place tray in oven and bake for 15 minutes.
7. Let dish cool down for 4-6 minutes and serve.

Nutrition per Serving: Calories - 269, Carbs - 4g, Fat – 20.9g, Protein - 18.45g

Baked Cauliflower Casserole

Prep time: 15 minutes | Cook time: 35 minutes | Servings: 4

Ingredients:

10 oz cauliflower, divided into small florets

½ tsp salt

1 tsp ground black pepper

4 eggs, beaten

1/3 cup coconut milk

2 tsp butter

5 oz green beans

7 oz Parmesan cheese, grated

Directions:

1. In bowl, combine cauliflower florets with salt and black pepper.
2. In another bowl, whisk together eggs and coconut milk.
3. Grease baking form with butter and put cauliflower florets in it.
4. Place green beans on top.
5. Pour egg mixture over green beans and sprinkle with cheese.
6. Set oven to 365 F and heat it up.
7. Place dish in oven and bake for 30 minutes.
8. Let it cool briefly and serve it immediately.

Nutrition per Serving: Calories - 309, Carbs - 10g, Fat – 20.9g, Protein – 23.9g

Spicy Roasted Asparagus

Prep time: 15 minutes | Cook time: 17 minutes | Servings: 4

Ingredients:

10 oz asparagus, washed and chopped roughly

1 tsp salt

2 tsp thyme

1 tsp minced garlic

1 tsp oregano

4 tbsp butter

1 tbsp lemon juice

1 oz walnuts, crushed

½ cup chicken stock

Directions:

1. In medium bowl, combine asparagus, salt, thyme, garlic, and oregano.
2. Preheat pan on medium high heat and melt butter.
3. Add lemon juice and bring liquid to boil.
4. Add crushed walnuts, stir.
5. Add asparagus and pour chicken stock. Stir well.
6. Close lid and simmer for 10 minutes on medium heat, until asparagus is soft.
7. Remove excess liquid from pan and serve dish.

Nutrition per Serving: Calories - 129, Carbs - 3.68g, Fat - 13g, Protein - 3g

Mixed Vegetable Dish

Prep time: 15 minutes | Cook time: 12 minutes | Servings: 4

Ingredients:

6 tbsp olive oil

2 tbsp garlic, minced

14 oz mushrooms, sliced

3 oz broccoli florets

3 oz bell pepper, seeded and cut into strips

½ cup sugar snap peas

Salt and ground black pepper to taste

A pinch of red pepper flakes

2 tbsp pumpkin seeds

3 oz spinach, torn

Directions:

1. Preheat pan with olive oil on medium high heat.
2. Add garlic and stir. Sauté for 1 minute.
3. Put mushrooms in pan, stir. Sauté for 3 minutes more.
4. Add broccoli and stir again.
5. Add bell pepper and snap peas, stir gently.
6. Season with black pepper, salt and pepper flakes.
7. Add pumpkin seeds. Stir and cook for 3-4 minutes.
8. Add spinach and stir mixture carefully. Cook for 2-3 minutes.
9. Let dish cool down for few minutes and serve warm.

Nutrition per Serving: Calories - 250, Carbs – 2.9g, Fat – 22.9g, Protein – 6.96g

Delicious Stuffed Eggs

Prep time: 5 minutes | Cook time: 0 minutes | Servings: 4

Ingredients:

6 eggs, boiled and peeled

6 bacon strips, cooked and chopped

1/3 tsp cayenne pepper

1½ tsp dill

1/3 cup cream cheese

3 oz Parmesan cheese, grated

½ tsp salt

Directions:

1. Cut eggs in half.
2. In medium bowl, combine bacon, cayenne pepper and dill.
3. In another bowl, mix together cream cheese and Parmesan cheese.
4. Add cheese mixture to bacon mixture and stir well. Season with salt.
5. Take out egg yolks from eggs and put them in bacon mixture.
6. Fill egg whites with this mixture and serve.

Nutrition per Serving: Calories - 250, Carbs - 1.95g, Fat - 20g, Protein – 15.98g

Fried Cheese Sticks

Prep time: 10 minutes | Cook time: 5 minutes | Servings: 2

Ingredients:

2 large eggs, beaten

1 tbsp flax seeds

1 tsp basil

¼ tsp salt

½ tsp chili flakes

1 tsp oregano

4 tbsp butter

4 oz Cheddar cheese, cut into thick strips

Directions:

1. In medium bowl, whisk eggs until get homogenous mass.
2. In small bowl, mix together flax seeds, basil, salt, chili flakes, and oregano.
3. Heat up pan over medium high heat and melt butter.
4. Dip Cheddar sticks in egg mixture and season them with spice mixture.
5. Toss stick on pan and fry for 1 minute per each side or until crispy.
6. Transfer to paper towels and remove excess fat.
7. Serve.

Nutrition per Serving: Calories - 530, Carbs - 2.57g, Fat - 49g, Protein – 20.9g

Tender Pumpkin Side Dish

Prep time: 10 minutes | Cook time: 12 minutes | Servings: 4

Ingredients:

8 oz pumpkin puree

5 tbsp chicken stock

1 tbsp almond milk

½ tsp dried oregano

½ tsp dried basil

1 tsp kosher salt

1 tsp ground paprika

1 tbsp chia seeds

¼ cup pumpkin seeds, crushed

Directions:

1. Start to preheat pan on medium heat.
2. In pan, combine pumpkin puree, chicken stock and almond milk.
3. Stirring pumpkin mass frequently, bring to boil.
4. Sprinkle with oregano, basil, salt, paprika and chia seeds.
5. Cook for 5 minutes, stirring constantly.
6. Let pumpkin puree cool down for few minutes.
7. Season with crushed pumpkin seeds and serve.

Nutrition per Serving: Calories - 111, Carbs – 7.98g, Fat - 7.9g, Protein - 4.53g

Mushroom and Hemp Pilaf

Prep time: 15 minutes | Cook time: 25 minutes | Servings: 4

Ingredients:

2 tbsp butter

3 mushrooms, chopped

2 oz almonds, sliced

1 cup hemp seeds

½ cup chicken stock

½ tsp garlic powder

Salt and ground black pepper to taste

¼ tsp dried parsley

Directions:

1. Preheat pan on medium heat and melt butter.
2. Put mushrooms and almond in pan and stir. Sauté for 4 minutes.
3. Add hemp seeds and stir again.
4. Pour in chicken stock.
5. Add garlic powder, black pepper, salt and parsley. Stir well.
6. Close lid and simmer on low heat until liquid is absorbed.
7. Serve warm.

Nutrition per Serving: Calories - 319, Carbs – 1.95g, Fat – 23.9g, Protein – 14.87g

Stuffed Mushrooms

Prep time: 12 minutes | Cook time: 25 minutes | Servings: 4

Ingredients:

1 medium onion

1 cup shrimp, cooked

¼ cup mayonnaise

¼ cup sour cream

1 tsp garlic powder

4 oz cream cheese, softened

1 tsp curry powder

½ cup Queso Blanco or Monterey Jack cheese, shredded

Salt and ground black pepper to taste

24 oz white mushroom caps

Directions:

1. Peel and chop onion.
2. Peel, devein and chop shrimp.
3. In mixing bowl, combine mayonnaise, sour cream, garlic powder, cream cheese, onion, and curry powder. Stir well.
4. Add shrimp and Queso Blanco cheese, stir.
5. Sprinkle with salt and pepper to taste.
6. Preheat oven to 350 F.
7. Stuff mushrooms with cheese mixture and place on baking sheet.
8. Bake in oven for about 20 minutes.
9. Serve warm..

Nutrition per Serving: Calories - 250, Carbs – 6.9g, Fat – 19.8g, Protein – 13.9g

Sweet Strawberry Side Dish

Prep time: 15 minutes | Cook time: 22 minutes | Servings: 5

Ingredients:

2 tbsp almond milk

1 tbsp Almond flour

1 tbsp butter

½ cup ground chicken

¼ tsp ground black pepper

7 oz avocado, pitted and peeled

1 cup strawberries, washed and chopped

5 tbsp water

1 white onion, peeled and diced

1 tsp stevia

1 cup lettuce, chopped roughly

Directions:

1. In mixing bowl, mixt together almond milk and almond flour. Stir, until get homogenous consistency.
2. Preheat pan on medium heat and melt butter.
3. Toss ground chicken with black pepper in pan and stir.
4. Cover pan and cook meat for 5 minutes.
5. Meanwhile, mash avocado with fork and add to almond mixture. Mix up well.
6. Add strawberries and stir.
7. Add this mixture to pan and stir.
8. Pour in water and add onion and stevia. Stir well.
9. Close lid and cook for 10 minutes.
10. Let mixture cool down for 2 minutes and add lettuce.
11. Serve warm.

Nutrition per Serving: Calories - 159, Carbs – 7.9g, Fat – 13.1g, Protein – 5.67g

Healthy Stuffed Mushrooms

Prep time: 15 minutes | Cook time: 12 minutes | Servings: 4

Ingredients:

1 clove garlic

8 oz parsley

4 oz sundried tomatoes

4 oz cup pine nuts

¼ tsp sea salt

1 tsp lemon juice

¼ cup extra virgin olive oil

8 oz mushrooms caps

Directions:

1. Chop garlic and parsley.
2. Place parsley in blender or food processor and blend.
3. Put garlic, tomatoes, pine nuts, and salt in food processor.
4. Pour in lemon juice and blend until smooth.
5. Pour in olive oil and blend well.
6. Stuff mushrooms caps with this sauce.
7. Preheat oven to 350 F and bake stuffed mushrooms for 10 minutes.
8. Serve warm.

Nutrition per Serving: Calories – 269, Carbs - 9g, Fat - 27g, Protein: 5.51g

Creamy Pecan Balls

Prep time: 20 minutes | Cook time: 8 minutes | Servings: 3

Ingredients:

½ cup pecan, cut in half

1 tsp coconut oil

¼ cup cream cheese

1 tbsp butter

½ tsp dried basil

1 tsp dried dill

Directions:

1. Set oven to 360 F and heat it up.
2. Place pecan halves on baking sheet, sprinkle with coconut oil and put in oven.
3. Cook for 6 minutes. Then, let them cool down.
4. In medium bowl, combine cream cheese and butter. Mix until smooth.
5. Season with basil and dill, stir.
6. Spread each pecan halves with cheese mixture and fridge for 5-10 minutes.
7. Serve.

Nutrition per Serving: Calories - 381, Carbs – 5.98g, Fat - 40g, Protein - 5.75g

Green Beans with Vinaigrette

Prep time: 15 minutes | Cook time: 15 minutes | Servings: 8

Ingredients:

1 garlic clove

2 oz chorizo

¼ tsp coriander

Salt and ground black pepper to taste

2 tsp smoked paprika

½ cup coconut vinegar

1 tsp lemon juice

2 tbsp beef stock

4 tbsp macadamia nut oil

2 tbsp coconut oil

2 pound green beans

Directions:

1. Peel and chop garlic. Chop chorizo.
2. Place garlic, chorizo, coriander, black pepper, salt, paprika, coconut vinegar, and lemon juice in blender or food processor and blend well.
3. Pour in beef stock, add macadamia nut oil and pulse again.
4. Preheat pan on medium heat and add coconut oil.
5. Toss green beans and chorizo mixture in pan and cook for 10 minutes, stirring occasionally.
6. Serve.

Nutrition per Serving: Calories - 158, Carbs – 5.95g, Fat – 11.9g, Protein – 4.11g

Egg Chips

Prep time: 15 minutes | Cook time: 17 minutes | Servings: 3

Ingredients:

4 medium eggs, beaten

½ tsp ground black pepper

A pinch of salt

3 oz Cheddar cheese, grated

1 tsp butter

Directions:

1. In medium bowl, whisk eggs with black pepper and salt.
2. Prepare muffin forms. Fill each form with 1 tablespoon of egg mixture.
3. Put grated cheese on top of mixture.
4. Set oven to 350 F and heat it up.
5. Place muffin forms in oven and bake dish for 15 minutes.
6. Let chips cool briefly and serve.

Nutrition per Serving: Calories - 309, Carbs - 1.75g, Fat - 25g, Protein - 22g

Keto Zucchini Noodles

Prep time: 10 minutes | Cook time: 12 minutes | Servings: 4

Ingredients:

2 zucchini, washed

8 oz chicken stock

½ tsp cayenne pepper

½ tsp paprika

¼ cup cream cheese

1 tsp butter

1 oz olives, pitted and sliced

1 tsp sea salt

Directions:

1. With help of spiralizer, make noodles from zucchini.
2. Pour stock in saucepan and heat it up over medium heat.
3. Season with paprika, cayenne pepper, and salt.
4. Bring chicken stock to boil and add zucchini noodles.
5. Cover saucepan and cook for 4 minutes.
6. Transfer noodles to mixing bowl and add cream cheese. Stir carefully.
7. Add butter and olives, stir carefully.
8. Serve.

Nutrition per Serving: Calories - 70, Carbs - 3.85g, Fat - 5.87g, Protein - 2.2g

Creamy Asparagus

Prep time: 12 minutes | Cook time: 17 minutes | Servings: 3

Ingredients:

10 oz asparagus spears

2 oz cream cheese

⅓ cup heavy cream

2 tbsp mustard

⅓ cup Monterey jack cheese, shredded

2 tbsp Parmesan cheese, grated

3 tbsp bacon, cooked

Salt and ground black pepper to taste

Directions:

1. Cut asparagus into medium-sized pieces and steam.
2. Put cream cheese, heavy cream and mustard in pan, stir well.
3. Heat up pan over medium heat, stirring mixture occasionally.
4. Add Parmesan cheese and Monterey Jack cheese, stir well and cook until it melts.
5. Crumble bacon and add 1½ tablespoon to pan.
6. Add asparagus, stir and cook for 3 minutes more.
7. Add remaining bacon and sprinkle with salt and black pepper, stir.
8. Cook for 5 minutes more.
9. Serve warm.

Nutrition per Serving: Calories - 260, Carbs – 4.93g, Fat – 22.9g, Protein – 12.8g

Cheddar Bites

Prep time: 15 minutes | Cook time: 17 minutes | Servings: 4

Ingredients:

8 oz Cheddar cheese, grated

½ tsp ground black pepper

1 tsp salt

2 large eggs, beaten

1 tsp basil

1 tsp dill

2 oz almond flour

2 oz cream

2 oz walnuts, crushed

1 tbsp butter

Directions:

1. In medium bowl, mix together Cheddar cheese, black pepper and salt.
2. In another bowl, whisk eggs.
3. Pour whisked eggs in cheese mixture. Sprinkle with basil and dill.
4. Add almond flour and cream, mix well.
5. Add nuts and stir again.
6. Set oven to 360 F and heat it up.
7. Grease baking sheet with butter.
8. Shape mixture into cheese balls 1½-inch in diameter and put on baking sheet.
9. Place balls in oven and cook for 15 minutes.
10. Let dish cool down for few minutes and serve.

Nutrition per Serving: Calories – 338g, Carbs - 3.65g, Fat - 30g, Protein - 18g

Raspberry and Coconut Dessert

Prep time: 15 minutes | Cook time: 7 minutes | Servings: 10

Ingredients:

4 oz cup dried raspberries

4 oz cup coconut butter

¼ cup swerve

½ cup coconut oil

4 oz cup coconut, shredded

Directions:

1. Place raspberries in blender or food processor and blend well.
2. Preheat pan on medium heat and melt butter.
3. Pour in swerve and coconut oil. Add shredded coconut, stir and cook for 5 minutes.
4. Pour half coconut mixture into lined baking pan and spread well.
5. Sprinkle with raspberry powder. Then top with remaining coconut mixture.
6. Place in refrigerator for 2-3 hours.
7. Cut into pieces and serve.

Nutrition per Serving: Calories - 229, Carbs – 3.96g, Fat – 21.9g, Protein – 2.15g

Crispy Pecan Bars

Prep time: 20 minutes | Cook time: 35 minutes | Servings: 6

Ingredients:

2 tbsp almond flour

1 cup butter

1 cup coconut flour

1 tsp vanilla extract

2 egg yolks

25 drops Stevia

3 oz pecans, crushed

1 oz dark chocolate

Directions:

1. In medium bowl, mix together almond flour, butter and coconut flour.
2. Add vanilla extract, egg yolks, and stevia. Stir well.
3. Add crushed pecans and mix up well.
4. Knead non-sticky dough with help of your hands.
5. Set oven to 365 F and heat it up.
6. Roll dough and cut in 2 x 1" pieces.
7. Place pieces on baking sheet lined with parchment paper and put in oven.
8. Bake for 15 minutes.
9. In saucepan, melt dark chocolate on low heat.
10. When cookies are cooked, let them cool down for few minutes.
11. Spread melted chocolate on cookies and set aside for 1-2 minutes.
12. Serve.

Nutrition per Serving: Calories - 391, Carbs - 6g, Fat – 40.1g, Protein - 4g

Chocolate Cups

Prep time: 35 minutes | Cook time: 7 minutes | Servings: 18

Ingredients:

½ cup coconut oil

4 oz coconut butter

¼ cup swerve + 3 tbsp swerve

½ cup coconut, shredded

1 oz chocolate, unsweetened

1.5 oz cocoa butter

¼ tsp vanilla extract

¼ cup cocoa powder

Directions:

1. Preheat pan with oil on medium heat. Toss butter and melt it.
2. Add 3 tablespoons swerve and shredded coconut, stir.
3. Transfer coconut mixture to lined muffins pan.
4. Place in refrigerator for 30 minutes.
5. In medium bowl, combine chocolate, cocoa butter, ¼ cup swerve, vanilla extract, and cocoa powder. Mix well.
6. Place this mixture over bowl filled with boiling water and stir until chocolate is melted and mixture is smooth.
7. Spread chocolate mixture over coconut cupcakes and place in refrigerator for 15-20 minutes.
8. Serve.

Nutrition per Serving: Calories - 239, Carbs – 4.8g, Fat – 24g, Protein – 1.95g

Green Vanilla Pudding

Prep time: 20 minutes | Cook time: 7 minutes | Servings: 4

Ingredients:

7 oz avocado, pitted, peeled and chopped roughly

8 oz almond milk

1 tsp Erythritol

1 tsp lemon juice

1 tsp vanilla extract

2 tbsp stevia

Directions:

1. Put avocado in blender or food processor and blend until smooth.
2. Pour almond milk in blender and blend for another 2 minutes.
3. Add Erythritol, lemon juice, vanilla extract, and stevia. Blend for 30 seconds.
4. Keep mixture in freezer for 5 minutes.
5. Remove pudding from freezer and divide between serving glasses.
6. Serve.

Nutrition per Serving: Calories - 239, Carbs - 8g, Fat – 23.9g, Protein - 3.65g

Berry Mousse

Prep time: 12 minutes | Cook time: 0 minutes | Servings: 10

Ingredients:

8 oz mascarpone cheese

¾ tsp stevia

1 cup whipping cream

½ tsp vanilla extract

½ pint strawberries

½ pint blueberries

Directions:

1. Combine mascarpone, stevia, vanilla extract and whipping cream.
2. Use hand mixer to blend mixture well.
3. Prepare 12 serving glasses.
4. Put layer of strawberries and blueberries in each glass.
5. Then put layer of cream mixture and so on.
6. Keep in refrigerator for 10-15 minutes.
7. Serve.

Nutrition per Serving: Calories – 145.5, Carbs – 2.98g, Fat – 11.9g, Protein – 1.98g

Lemon Mousse

Prep time: 12 minutes | Cook time: 0 minutes | Servings: 5

Ingredients:

8 oz mascarpone cheese

8 oz heavy cream

½ cup lemon juice

¼ tsp kosher salt

1 tsp stevia

Directions:

1. Using hand mixer, combine together mascarpone, heavy cream and lemon juice.
2. Sprinkle with salt and stevia. Mix up mixture again.
3. Prepare serving glasses.
4. Spread mousse in glasses and place in refrigerator at least for 15 minutes.
5. Serve.

Nutrition per Serving: Calories - 270, Carbs – 1.98g, Fat – 26.9g, Protein – 3.95g

Gingerbread Cookies

Prep time: 20 minutes | Cook time: 12 minutes | Servings: 5

Ingredients:

1 tsp ground ginger

1 cup almond flour

1 tsp cinnamon

1 tsp cardamom

1 tsp vanilla extract

½ tsp baking soda

3 medium eggs, beaten

5 tbsp butter, softened

50 drops stevia

1 tbsp lemon juice

Directions:

1. In medium bowl, mix together ground ginger, almond flour, cinnamon, cardamom, vanilla, and baking soda.
2. Add eggs and stir well, preferably using hand mixer.
3. Then add butter and continue to whisk dough.
4. Add lemon juice and stevia, stir again.
5. Knead the dough with your hands and keep it in fridge for 10-15 minutes.
6. Set oven to 350 F and heat it up.
7. Roll out the chilled cookie dough discs until about 1/4-inch thick.
8. Form (or cut) gingerbread men from dough.
9. Line baking sheet with parchment paper.
10. Place cookies onto lined baking sheet about 1 inch apart.
11. Put in oven and bake for about 10-12 minutes.
12. Let cookies cool completely. Serve.

Nutrition per Serving: Calories - 151, Carbs – 2.25g, Fat – 13.97g, Protein – 3.9g

Peanut Butter and Chocolate Brownies

Prep time: 15 minutes | Cook time: 35 minutes | Servings: 4

Ingredients:

7 tbsp butter

⅓ cup Erythritol

⅓ cup cocoa powder

¼ tsp salt

½ tsp vanilla extract

1 big egg, beaten

¼ cup almond flour

½ tsp baking powder

¼ cup walnuts, crushed

1 tbsp peanut butter

Directions:

1. Preheat pan on medium heat, add 6 tablespoons butter and melt it. Add Erythritol, stir and cook for 5 minutes.
2. Transfer butter mixture to medium bowl and add cocoa powder, salt, and vanilla extract, mix up well.
3. Add egg and whisk mixture.
4. Add almond flour, baking powder and walnuts. Mix well.
5. Transfer this mixture to baking pan.
6. In small heatproof bowl, combine peanut butter with 1 tablespoon butter.
7. Heat bowl slightly to melt butter.
8. Spread butter mixture over brownies mixture in pan.
9. Preheat oven to 350 F.
10. Put in oven and bake for 30 minutes.
11. Remove brownies from oven and set aside to cool.
12. Cut and serve.

Nutrition per Serving: Calories - 228, Carbs – 2.98g, Fat – 31.9g, Protein – 5.9g

Delicious Chocolate Peanut Butter Muffins

Prep time: 25 minutes | Cook time: 32 minutes | Servings: 3

Ingredients:

1 cup almond flour

1 tsp baking powder

¼ tsp salt

½ cup erythritol

1/3 cup peanut butter, softened

1/3 cup almond milk

2 large eggs, beaten

½ cup cacao nibs (or sugar-free chocolate chips)

Directions:

1. In medium bowl, mix together almond flour, baking powder, salt and erythritol.
2. Add butter and stir well.
3. Pour in almond milk and stir.
4. Add eggs and mix well.
5. Toss cacao nibs and stir mixture gently.
6. Grease 12 muffin molds with cooking spray and fill them with batter.
7. Preheat oven to 350 F.
8. Place in oven and bake for 15 minutes.
9. Serve.

Nutrition per 2 Muffins: Calories – 527, Carbs – 4.4g, Fat – 40.8g, Protein – 14.8g

Fast-Cook Grated Pie

Prep time: 20 minutes | Cook time: 35 minutes | Servings: 5

Ingredients:

1 egg, beaten

5 tbsp butter, softened

4 oz coconut flour

1 tsp Erythritol

8 oz almond flour

4 oz raspberries

1 tbsp stevia extract

Directions:

1. In medium bowl, whisk together egg and butter until get homogenous consistency.
2. Add coconut flour and Erythritol. Mix up mixture.
3. Sprinkle almond flour and knead dough with your hands.
4. In small bowl, mash raspberries with fork and add stevia extract. Stir well.
5. Halve dough into 2 parts.
6. Put dough in fridge at least for 30 minutes.
7. Line baking sheet with parchment paper.
8. Remove dough from fridge and grate 1 half on parchment paper.
9. Spread raspberry mixture on grated dough.
10. Then grate second half of dough.
11. Set oven to 365 F and heat it up.
12. Put baking sheet in oven and bake for 25-30 minutes.
13. Let pie cool for few minutes and serve.

Nutrition per Serving: Calories - 211, Carbs - 6.65g, Fat - 20g, Protein - 3.65g

Mug Cake

Prep time: 5 minutes | Cook time: 2 minutes | Servings: 1

Ingredients:

2 tbsp butter, melted

½ tsp baking powder

1 medium egg, beaten

1 tbsp cocoa powder, unsweetened

1 tbsp coconut flour

¼ tsp vanilla extract

1 tsp stevia

4 tbsp almond meal

Directions:

1. In mug, combine melted butter, baking powder, egg, cocoa powder, coconut flour, stevia, and vanilla. Mix well.
2. Add almond meal and stir.
3. Place mug in microwave and cook for about 2 minutes.
4. Serve warm.

Nutrition per Serving: Calories - 448, Carbs – 9.9g, Fat – 33.8g, Protein – 19.8g

Keto Soufflé

Prep time: 30 minutes | Cook time: 15 minutes | Servings: 4

Ingredients:

3 egg whites

1 tbsp cocoa powder

2 tbsp stevia extract

2 tbsp butter

1 tsp vanilla extract

1 oz dark chocolate

1 tbsp lemon juice

½ tsp baking powder

1 egg yolk

5 tbsp coconut milk

1 cup almond flour

Directions:

1. In bowl, whip egg whites with help of electric beaters or a standing mixer, on medium speed, till you get firm peaks.
2. Add cocoa powder and stevia and keep beating egg mixture for another 30 seconds.
3. Add butter and vanilla; continue to whip for 15 second.
4. Melt dark chocolate.
5. In bowl, mix chocolate with lemon juice and baking powder.
6. Add egg yolks and stir mixture until get homogenous mass.
7. Pour yolk egg mixture in egg white mixture and stir well.
8. Pour in coconut milk. Add almond flour.
9. Knead smooth liquid dough.
10. Prepare ramekins. Fill each ramekin halfway with dough.
11. Set oven to 375 F and heat it up.
12. Place ramekins in oven and cook for 15 minutes.
13. Serve hot.

Nutrition per Serving: Calories - 211, Carbs - 8.5g, Fat - 18g, Protein – 5.95g

Mixed Berries and Cream

Prep time: 10 minutes | Cook time: 0 minutes | Servings: 4

Ingredients:

1 and 2/3 cups heavy cream

3 tbsp cocoa powder

2 tbsp stevia

Coconut chips

8 oz raspberries

8 oz blackberries

Directions:

1. Combine heavy cream, cocoa powder and stevia. Mix up well.
2. Pour ½ part mixture in serving bowl and add coconut chips, raspberries and blackberries.
3. Then spread another part of mixture.
4. Top with berries and coconut chips.
5. Serve.

Nutrition per Serving: Calories - 238, Carbs – 5.9g, Fat – 33.7g, Protein – 1.98g

Sweet Bombs

Prep time: 15 minutes | Cook time: 17 minutes | Servings: 4

Ingredients:

2 eggs, beaten

½ tsp vanilla extract

2 tbsp Erythritol

½ cup coconut, shredded

1 cup almond flour

1 tbsp butter, softened

Directions:

1. In medium bowl, whip eggs with help of electric beaters or hand whisker.
2. Add vanilla and Erythritol, stir well.
3. Add coconut and almond flour, knead dough.
4. Add butter and mix until get homogenous and smooth mass.
5. Set oven to 360 F and heat it up.
6. Line baking sheet with parchment paper.
7. Make small sweet bombs from dough and put them on baking sheet.
8. Place in oven and cook sweet bombs for 15 minutes.
9. When dessert is cooked, let it cool down and serve.

Nutrition per Serving: Calories - 198, Carbs – 5.95g, Fat – 17.9g, Protein - 5.4g

Chocó Peanut Butter Milkshake

Prep time: 7 minutes | Cook time: 0 minutes | Servings: 1

Ingredients:

1 cup unsweetened coconut milk

1 tbsp unsweetened cocoa powder

1 tbsp natural peanut butter

1 scoop protein powder

1 tsp liquid stevia

¼ tsp sea salt

Directions:

1. Place coconut milk, cocoa powder, peanut butter, protein powder, stevia and salt in blender or food processor and blend until texture is smooth.
2. Serve.

Nutrition per Serving: Calories – 334, Carbs – 9.8g, Fat - 36g, Protein – 16.7g

Chocolate Fluffy Pie

Prep time: 30 minutes | Cook time: 14 minutes | Servings: 4

Ingredients:

1 large egg, beaten

1 tbsp almond milk

1 tsp Erythritol

1 cup coconut flour

1 tsp baking powder

4 tbsp butter, softened

1 tbsp lemon juice

½ cup cream

1 cup cream cheese

1 tsp cocoa

4 tsp stevia extract

Directions:

1. In medium bowl, whip eggs. Add almond milk and Erythtitol and continue to whip.
2. Add coconut flour, baking powder and butter and mix up mixture.
3. Pour in lemon juice and knead dough.
4. Line baking pan with parchment paper and pour dough in it.
5. Set oven to 370 F and heat it up.
6. Prick dough with fork and place baking pan in oven.
7. Bake pie for 12 minutes.
8. In bowl, whip cream with hand whisker until get fluffy mass.
9. Add cream cheese and whip mixture again until get smooth and soft texture.
10. Add cocoa and stevia, stir mass gently.
11. Put this mixture in fridge.
12. When pie is cooked, let it cool down.
13. Spread cocoa cream mixture over pie and keep pie in fridge for 10 minutes.
14. Serve.

Nutrition per Serving: Calories - 209, Carbs – 3.47g, Fat – 25.9g, Protein – 7.9g

Almond-Strawberry Smoothie

Prep time: 12 minutes | Cook time: 0 minutes | Servings: 3

Ingredients:

17 oz unsweetened almond milk

¼ cup frozen strawberries

1 scoop vegetarian protein powder

3.5 oz heavy cream

Stevia to taste

Directions:

1. Place strawberries and almond milk in blender or food processor and blend well.
2. Add heavy cream, protein powder and stevia, continue blend until mass is smooth.
3. Serve.

Nutrition per Serving: Calories – 311, Carbs – 6.9g, Fat - 24g, Protein – 14.8g

Keto Blackberry Muffins

Prep time: 15 minutes | Cook time: 22 minutes | Servings: 4

Ingredients:

1 cup almond flour

1 tsp baking soda

1 oz dark chocolate, melted

4 oz blackberries

4 oz almond milk

1 tbsp stevia extract

1 tbsp apple cider vinegar

Directions:

1. In medium bowl, mix together almond flour and baking soda.
2. Add dark chocolate and stir.
3. In another bowl, mash blackberries with spoon.
4. Pour in almond milk and stir mixture until get homogenous mass.
5. Pour this mixture into almond flour mixture and stir well.
6. Add vinegar and stevia extract. Stir mixture until get smooth dough.
7. Set oven to 350 F and heat it up.
8. Prepare silicon muffin molds and fill ½ of every form with dough.
9. Place muffins in oven and bake for 20 minutes.
10. Let muffins cool briefly and remove them from silicon forms.
11. Serve immediately.

Nutrition per Serving: Calories - 120, Carbs - 7.74g, Fat - 9.45g, Protein - 1.48g

Pineapple Smoothie

Prep time: 7 minutes | Cook time: 1 minutes | Servings: 1

Ingredients:

18 blanched almonds

4 oz plain yogurt

½ cup almond milk

2 oz fresh or frozen pineapple pieces

Directions:

1. Place almonds, yogurt, almond milk and pineapple in food processor or blender and blend until get smooth mass.
2. Toss ice cubes in mixture to get cooler smoothie, if desired.

Nutrition per Serving: Calories – 277, Carbs – 16.8g, Fat - 19g, Protein - 11g

Vanilla Gelatin Cake

Prep time: 2 hours | Cook time: 25 minutes | Servings: 3

Ingredients:

8 oz almond milk

8 oz cream

5 tbsp water

3 tbsp gelatin powder

2 tbsp stevia extract

1 tsp vanilla extract

1 tsp cinnamon

Directions:

1. In saucepan, mix together almond milk and cream.
2. Heat up saucepan over low heat, until almond mixture is warm.
3. In another saucepan boil water and remove from heat. Add gelatin and stir until dissolved.
4. Sprinkle vanilla extract and stevia extract, stir carefully until get homogenous consistency.
5. Then pour gelatin mixture in almond mixture and whip it thoroughly, until smooth.
6. Add cinnamon and stir again.
7. Stirring occasionally, bring this mixture to boil on medium heat and remove from heat.
8. Let mixture cool for 3-5 minutes and transfer to silicon mold.
9. Keep cake in freeze for 2 hours.
10. Serve.

Nutrition per Serving: Calories - 340, Carbs - 8g, Fat – 24.1g, Protein – 27.2g

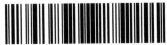

61817209R00113

Made in the USA
Middletown, DE
21 August 2019